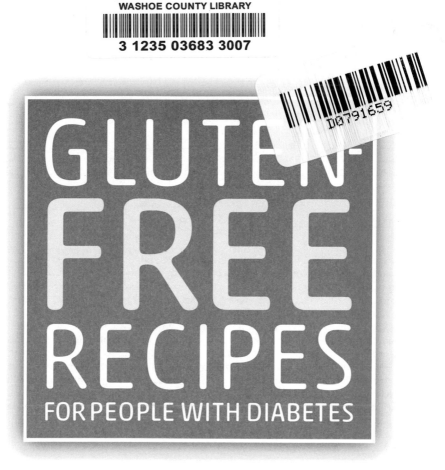

GLUTEN-FREE RECIPES

FOR PEOPLE WITH DIABETES

NANCY S. HUGHES

INTRODUCTION BY
LARA RONDINELLI-HAMILTON, RD, LDN, CDE

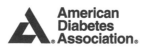

American Diabetes Association.

Director, Book Publishing, Abe Ogden; *Managing Editor,* Greg Guthrie; *Acquisitions Editor,* Victor Van Beuren; *Production Manager,* Melissa Sprott; *Composition,* Naylor Design, Inc.; *Cover Design,* Jody Billert; *Printer,* United Graphics, Inc.

Printed in the United States of America
1 3 5 7 9 10 8 6 4 2

The suggestions and information contained in this publication are generally consistent with the *Clinical Practice Recommendations* and other policies of the American Diabetes Association, but they do not represent the policy or position of the Association or any of its boards or committees. Reasonable steps have been taken to ensure the accuracy of the information presented. However, the American Diabetes Association cannot ensure the safety or efficacy of any product or service described in this publication. Individuals are advised to consult a physician or other appropriate health care professional before undertaking any diet or exercise program or taking any medication referred to in this publication. Professionals must use and apply their own professional judgment, experience, and training and should not rely solely on the information contained in this publication before prescribing any diet, exercise, or medication. The American Diabetes Association—its officers, directors, employees, volunteers, and members—assumes no responsibility or liability for personal or other injury, loss, or damage that may result from the suggestions or information in this publication.

∞ The paper in this publication meets the requirements of the ANSI Standard Z39.48-1992 (permanence of paper).

ADA titles may be purchased for business or promotional use or for special sales. To purchase more than 50 copies of this book at a discount, or for custom editions of this book with your logo, contact the American Diabetes Association at the address below, at booksales@diabetes.org, or by calling 703-299-2046.

American Diabetes Association
1701 North Beauregard Street
Alexandria, Virginia 22311

DOI: 10.2337/9781580404952

Library of Congress Cataloging-in-Publication Data

Hughes, Nancy S.
  Gluten-free recipes for people with diabetes / Nancy S. Hughes, Lara Rondinelli-Hamilton.
    pages cm
  Includes bibliographical references and index.
  ISBN 978-1-58040-495-2 (alk. paper)
  1. Diabetes--Diet therapy--Recipes. 2. Gluten-free diet--Recipes. I. Rondinelli-Hamilton, Lara, 1974- II. Title.
  RC662.H837 2013
  641.5'6314--dc23
                                                                                    2012049801

To my sister, Judy Wilcox. You carved your own path through trial and error sometimes, but you finally found a "safe" way to eat. I learned a lot from you, though (as the younger sister) I never really wanted to actually admit it! Thanks for being a great example of how someone who is seriously gluten intolerant can "savor the morsels" with total satisfaction! I love you, Judy!

—Nancy

Contents

Acknowledgments

Thank you to Abe Ogden, Director of Book Publishing, for asking me to be involved in this project. You are a true professional and have been wonderful to work with. Thank you to Nancy Hughes for helping everyone see the need for this book and for all your time and work put into creating the recipes. Thank you to Greg Guthrie for your expertise and help once again.

Thank you to Sue Mikolaitis, the dietitian that I saw when I was diagnosed with celiac disease. My specialty at that time was only diabetes and you taught me so much about the gluten-free world. Thank you to the University of Chicago Celiac Disease Center. You are a tremendous resource for all of us and your research is incredible. I'm so grateful for the Center and for all the wonderful people there including Dr. Guandalini, Carol Shilson, Ronit Rose, and Lara Field.

Thank you to all the food companies, restaurants, bakeries, and stores that offer gluten-free food and make our lives easier. I can't say thank you enough to my parents, sisters, mother and father-in-law, friends, and Dinner Club girls for making sure I always have something gluten-free to eat when I come to your house. You all have learned so much about gluten-free food and I appreciate all the care, work, and expense you put into having me over (and for always agreeing to eat at gluten-friendly restaurants). Thank you to my husband, Jared, for becoming a gluten-free expert and for always looking out for me and for telling restaurants, "You can't just take those croutons off the salad and bring it back to her; you have to make a new salad now." Jared—thank you for your love, support, feedback, editing skills, and for being a great dad and husband. And to my two little ones, Ethan and Penelope, thanks for making me laugh every day. I love you so much and I'm so proud of the little people you are becoming.

Finally, thank you to all my patients with celiac disease and diabetes who continue to inspire me every day. Thank you for sharing your stories with me. I hope this makes your gluten-free, diabetes life a little easier.

—*Lara Rondinelli-Hamilton RD,LDN,CDE*

I want to thank Abe Odgen for believing in me and listening to me, and in return, I listen to him and keep the readers' needs utmost in my mind and in my heart when I'm developing recipes for them.

Thanks also go to Greg Guthrie. Although we still have not met in person, I truly feel he is guiding me every step of the way! And thanks to you, Lara, for making sense of it all in a way that is not overwhelming. You provided awareness in laymen's terms!

Thanks to Melanie McKibbin, my multitasking business manager, who just found out she is gluten intolerant, ADORES good food, and is much happier and healthier now that she knows what she should avoid! To Wes Shepherd, my right arm, who makes sense of the crazy days, calms me down when I get a bit carried away, and is always, ALWAYS there when I need an extra hand . . . with a smile!

Thanks to my children: Will, Annie, and Taft, and their spouses: Kelly, Terry, and Kara, and my granddaughters: Jilli, Jesse, Emma, Molly Catherine, and Anna Flynn, who never ever know what's cooking, who's in the kitchen, who's shopping, chopping, and cleaning up . . . but they do know that they're loved to death no matter what's going on and there's always something good to eat . . . at all times!

And, finally, thanks to my husband, Greg . . . whew, I had no idea when we first started out that life would be this exciting, fun, adventurous, delicious, and . . . hilarious. Thanks for being there with me every single second!

—*Nancy S. Hughes*

Preface

MY STORY

In February 2007, I was biopsy diagnosed with celiac disease. My life changed dramatically with this diagnosis, as I now have to follow a strict gluten-free diet. I went from being a registered dietitian (RD) counseling patients on what to eat, to being the patient wondering what I could eat. I remember it vividly: sitting in my office and thinking that my Italian Christmas celebrations full of lasagna, eggplant Parmesan, biscotti, and cookies would never be the same. Even though I was an RD, I had a lot to learn about the gluten-free diet. My specialty was diabetes, so I knew much more about diabetes and healthy carbohydrates than celiac disease and gluten. Five years later, I've become very accustomed to eating gluten-free foods at home, restaurants, parties, and when traveling.

Historically, celiac disease has been an underdiagnosed disease, and although the awareness of the disease is increasing, there is still a lot more work to be done in this area. I believe I had the disease for seven years before getting the proper diagnosis, and although I saw many doctors for several issues, no one ever recommended that I get screened for celiac disease. My initial symptoms were vague and included fatigue, joint pain, and swelling. Looking back, I realize I felt better when I didn't eat bread and flour products, but I didn't think I could have celiac disease because I wasn't really sick and I didn't have classic gastrointestinal symptoms, such as diarrhea, vomiting, and weight loss. Fast forward several years later, and while I was working on my second cookbook, *The Healthy Carb Diabetes Cookbook,* I started feeling sick. I could barely eat or absorb any food and I had every classic gastrointestinal symptom, including weight loss. I was tired and weak. I knew there was something seriously wrong with me. I went to my doctor and asked to be tested for celiac disease. I often wonder if I hadn't asked to be screened for celiac disease if my doctor would have suggested it at that time.

After I began eating a gluten-free diet, I slowly felt much better and was on my way to good health. During these beginning stages, I wanted to try every new product on the market. I soon learned that my diet could be full of a lot of delicious, but unhealthy, gluten-free cookies, cakes, and treats. And, while I think we must be grateful for all gluten-free products that are available, a diet full of more natural foods, whole grains, lean protein, and fruits and vegetables is still the healthiest for all of us. A balanced diet is important for everyone and especially for those with diabetes and celiac disease.

Celiac disease is not as rare as people think. It is the most common inherited autoimmune disorder, and it affects about 1 of every 133 people in the U.S. (about 3 million Americans), with a marked predominance in non-Hispanic whites. Autoimmune thyroiditis, type 1 diabetes, Addison's disease, autoimmune liver disease, and Sjogren's syndrome occur more frequently in people with celiac disease. Many experts recommend that patients with these diseases be screened for celiac disease, whereas mass screening remains controversial. First-degree relatives to those with celiac disease should also be screened.

PURPOSE OF THIS GUIDE

People with diabetes have the double challenge of choosing foods that are gluten-free and diabetes-friendly. Many of the gluten-free mainstream products are low in fiber and high in refined carbohydrates that can elevate blood glucose levels. Eating and cooking healthfully with diabetes and celiac disease can be challenging, but it is possible. The American Diabetes Association (ADA) has recognized the need for a resource for people with diabetes and celiac disease.

The purpose of this introduction is to provide a resource of safe and healthy eating recommendations for those people with both diabetes and celiac disease. Nancy Hughes has created a wonderful cookbook consisting of delicious, healthy recipes suitable for people with both diabetes and celiac disease.

In addition to this guide, I've helped develop some healthy gluten-free, diabetes-friendly recipes on the ADA website.

Check out Recipes for Healthy Living, the American Diabetes Association's FREE online nutrition resource. Sign up today, and you'll get a sample meal plan, healthy tips, and a new set of recipes each month—with several quick and easy gluten-free dishes included! **Visit www.diabetes.org/recipes**

1

Celiac Disease and Diabetes

WHAT IS CELIAC DISEASE?

Celiac disease is an autoimmune disorder caused by eating gluten. It affects the digestive process of the small intestine. Gluten is a protein found in wheat, rye, and barley. When a person with celiac disease eats gluten, their immune system responds by attacking the small intestine and inhibits the absorption of nutrients into the body. Celiac disease is associated with other autoimmune disorders, such as type 1 diabetes and autoimmune thyroid disease. People with type 1 diabetes have a higher incidence of celiac disease, and it's estimated that 10% of people with type 1 diabetes (about 300,000 individuals) also have celiac disease. It is thought that untreated celiac disease may increase the risk of developing other autoimmune diseases.

People with celiac disease must avoid gluten entirely. Foods that contain gluten include anything with flour, such as bread, pasta, waffles, cookies, and cakes, but it's also hidden in foods, such as soy sauce, salad dressings, imitation crabmeat, some canned broth, and many more foods. For a complete list of foods that are safe and unsafe see pages 8–11.

SYMPTOMS OF CELIAC DISEASE

The symptoms of celiac disease can vary widely among individuals, and many people do NOT exhibit the traditional gastrointestinal symptoms, such as diarrhea. According to the University of Chicago Celiac Disease Center, common symptoms may include:

- Frequent abdominal bloating and pain
- Chronic diarrhea or constipation
- Vomiting
- Weight loss
- Pale, foul-smelling stool
- Iron-deficiency anemia that does not respond to iron therapy
- Fatigue
- Failure to thrive or short stature
- Delayed puberty
- Pain in the joints
- Tingling numbness in the legs
- Pale sores inside the mouth
- A skin rash called dermatitis herpetiformis
- Tooth discoloration or loss of enamel
- Unexplained infertility or recurrent miscarriage
- Osteopenia (mild) or osteoporosis (more serious bone density problem)
- Peripheral neuropathy
- Psychiatric disorders such as anxiety or depression

Interestingly, many people with type 1 diabetes who get diagnosed with celiac disease often do not have gastrointestinal symptoms or have minimal gastrointestinal symptoms. In addition, gastrointestinal symptoms are more common in children, and nongastrointestinal symptoms, such as anemia and osteoporosis, are more common in adults. Therefore, many experts state that you can't rely solely on gastrointestinal symptoms for diagnosis of celiac disease.

TYPE 1 DIABETES AND CELIAC DISEASE

People with type 1 diabetes or other autoimmune diseases are more at risk for celiac disease.

In an interview with Dr. Stefano Guandalini, an internationally recognized expert on celiac disease and medical director at the University of Chicago Celiac Disease Center, he explained the association between these diseases. According to Dr. Guandalini, certain autoimmune conditions share the same genetic predisposition. Type 1 diabetes and celiac disease share genetic similarities that increase their risks. In addition, Dr. Guandalini stated that there is evidence showing that untreated celiac disease and disturbed intestinal permeability (porous and allowing liquids to pass through) may open the pathway to other autoimmune conditions such as diabetes, Addison's disease, or thyroid disease. Most often, people are diagnosed with type 1 diabetes before celiac disease. This makes sense because type 1 diabetes can be the easier of the two to diagnose based on symptoms. The symptoms that present at type 1 diabetes diagnosis— excessive thirst, excessive urination, fatigue, and weight loss—can be easily recognized. Celiac disease symptoms vary among individuals and can include fatigue, joint pain, anemia, and diarrhea. Practitioners definitely have more experience in dealing with diabetes, but celiac disease awareness is increasing.

SCREENING AND DIAGNOSIS OF CELIAC DISEASE

Screening for celiac disease is done by a blood test to check for certain antibodies, specifically the tTG IgA. It's recommended that a person should be eating gluten for approximately 12 weeks prior to having this blood test done. A positive antibody test suggests that a person might have celiac disease, but multiple biopsies of the first portion of the small bowel are needed to diagnose celiac disease.

Screening Patients with Type 1 Diabetes for Celiac Disease
Below is the statement from the American Diabetes Association regarding screening recommendations for people with type 1 diabetes for celiac disease.

- Consider screening children with type 1 diabetes for celiac disease by measuring tissue transglutaminase or antiendomysial antibodies, with documentation of normal total serum IgA levels, soon after the diagnosis of diabetes.

- Testing should be considered in children with growth failure, failure to gain weight, weight loss, diarrhea, constipation, flatulence, abdominal pain, or signs of malabsorption, or in children with frequent unexplained hypoglycemia or deterioration in glycemic control.

- Consider referral to a gastroenterologist for evaluation with possible endoscopy and biopsy for confirmation of celiac disease in asymptomatic children with positive antibodies.

- Children with biopsy-confirmed celiac disease should be placed on a gluten-free diet and have consultation with a dietitian experienced in managing both diabetes and celiac disease.

WHAT IS THE TREATMENT FOR CELIAC DISEASE?

A strict, lifelong gluten-free diet is the treatment for celiac disease. A gluten-free diet will help alleviate symptoms and heal the damaged intestines. In most individuals, healing of the intestines can take anywhere from 6 to 24 months. If left untreated, celiac disease can lead to anemia, osteoporosis, lymphoma, vitamin and mineral deficiencies, depression, and infertility. The gluten-free diet is a lifelong treatment.

Does celiac diseases increase the risk for certain vitamin or mineral deficiencies?

Because celiac disease damages the small intestines, a person may not absorb nutrients properly, resulting in a higher risk of vitamin and mineral deficiencies. Iron, calcium, and vitamin D are the most common deficiencies, but some people have deficiencies in vitamin B12, copper, folic acid, magnesium, phosphorus, niacin, thiamine, riboflavin, or zinc. Various vitamin levels can be checked upon diagnosis of celiac disease. Due to the potential for deficiencies in calcium, vitamin D, and phosphorus, a bone density test (called a DEXA scan) should be considered to check for osteopenia and osteoporosis in adults and children with celiac disease. Talk to your doctor or RD about a multivitamin mineral supplement. Remember, all vitamins and medications must be checked to confirm gluten-free status.

2

Gluten-Free Diet 101

WHAT IS GLUTEN?

Gluten is a protein found in wheat, rye, and barley. Gluten is found in bread, pasta, cereal, crackers, soups, desserts, and many other foods. In addition, regular commercial oats are contaminated with gluten. Gluten is often a hidden ingredient in many foods, so it can be challenging to learn which foods contain gluten. People with celiac disease should see a dietitian who is specialized in the area. A person with diabetes and celiac disease would benefit from seeing a dietitian who ideally specializes in both. To find a dietitian specializing in celiac disease in your area, check out www.gluten-freedietitian.com and click on the link: "Dietitians Providing Counseling Services to Persons with Celiac Disease."

ARE OATS SAFE TO EAT IN A GLUTEN-FREE DIET?

Regular commercial oats are contaminated with gluten and should be avoided on a gluten-free diet. However, pure, uncontaminated oats can be consumed safely on a gluten-free diet up to a certain level.

Based on the totality of evidence conducted to date, *moderate amounts* of oats *not contaminated* with wheat, barley, or rye can be eaten on a daily basis by *most individuals* with celiac disease. The Academy of Nutrition and Dietetics Evidence Analysis Library states in part, "Studies have shown that incorporating oats uncontaminated with wheat, barley, or rye, into a gluten-free dietary pattern for people with celiac disease, at intake levels of approximately 50 grams dry oats per day, is generally safe and improves compliance."

When shopping for oats look for "gluten-free oats," "certified gluten-free oats," or "pure, uncontaminated oats." Some manufacturers of gluten-free oats include: Cream Hill Estates, Only Oats, Gluten-Free Oats, Bob's Red Mill, and Gifts of Nature. Adding gluten-free oats to your diet can significantly increase your fiber intake. Try adding them to the batter of pancakes, waffles, muffins, quick breads, and cookies.

It's important to note that under the Food Allergen Labeling Consumer Protection Act, if a food includes an ingredient that contains wheat protein, then the word "wheat" must be included on the label in either the ingredients list or a "Contains . . ." statement. In other words, simply look for the word "wheat," along with "barley," "malt," "rye," and "oats" (unless labeled gluten-free) to determine whether gluten is present.

Lists of ingredients to AVOID and SAFE ingredients from the University of Chicago Celiac Disease Center's *Jump Start Your Gluten-Free Diet* (2013) appear below and on pages 10–11.

Ingredients to Avoid (CONTAIN GLUTEN)

- Abyssinian Hard (Wheat Triticum duran)
- Avena (wild oat)
- Barley (Hordeum vulgare)
- Barley malt, barley extract
- Beer, ale, porter, stout, other fermented beverages
- Bleu Cheese**
- Bran
- Bread flour
- Broth**
- Bulgur (bulgur wheat and nuts)
- Bouillon
- Cereal (cereal extract, cereal binding)
- Cracker meal
- Croutons
- Couscous
- Dinkle***
- Durum***
- Einkorn, wild einkorn***
- Emmer, wild emmer***

- Edible starch
- Farina
- Farro***
- Filler
- Fu
- Flour (Including but not limited to: all-purpose, barley, bleached, bread, brown, durum, enriched, gluten, graham, granary, high protein, oat, wheat, white)
- Germ
- Gluten, Glutenin
- Graham flour
- Hordeum, Hordeum vulgare
- Hydrolyzed oat starch, hydrolyzed wheat gluten, hydrolyzed wheat protein
- Kamut***
- Malt, malt beverages, malt extract, malted milk, malt flavoring, malt syrup, malt vinegar, maltose
- Matzo (Matzah)
- MIR (wheat, rye)
- Miso (may contain barley)
- Mustard powder**
- Oats, oat bran, oat fiber, oat gum, oat syrup*
- Oriental wheat
- Rice malt, rice syrup, brown rice syrup**
- Rye
- Soy sauce**
- Seitan
- Semolina
- Spelt***
- Sprouted wheat
- Tabbuleh
- Triticale
- Udon
- Vital gluten
- Wheat, wheat berry, wheat bran, wheat germ, wheat germ oil, wheat grass, wheat gluten, wheat starch, whole wheat berries

* Historically, oats were not recommended because it was thought the avenin was toxic to gluten-intolerant individuals. However, research in Europe and the U.S. has found that oats are well tolerated by most people when consumed in moderation and do not contribute to abdominal symptoms, nor prevent intestinal healing. PLEASE NOTE: regular, commercially available oats are frequently contaminated with wheat or barely. However, "pure, uncontaminated" oats have become available from several companies in the U.S. and Canada. These companies process oats in dedicated facilities and are tested for purity. Pure, uncontaminated oats can be consumed safely in quantities of less than 1 cup per day. It is important that you talk to your physician and your registered dietitian prior to starting oats.
** May be made with wheat—call company to verify.
*** Types of wheat

Gluten-Free Ingredients (SAFE)

- Acorn
- Almond
- Amaranth
- Arborio rice
- Aromatic rice
- Arrowroot
- Basmati rice
- Brown rice, Brown rice flour
- Buckwheat
- Calrose
- Canola
- Cassava
- Channa
- Chestnut
- Chickpea
- Corn, corn flour, corn gluten, cornmeal, cornstarch
- Cottonseed
- Dal
- Dasheen flour
- Enriched rice
- Fava bean
- Flax, flax seeds
- Garbanzo
- Glutinous rice
- Hominy
- Instant rice
- Job's tears
- Millet
- Modified corn starch
- Modified tapioca starch
- Montina™
- Peanut flour
- Potato flour, potato starch
- Quinoa
- Red rice
- Rice, rice bran, rice flour
- Risotto
- Sago
- Sesame
- Sorghum
- Soy, soybean, tofu (soya)
- Starch (made from safe grains)
- Sunflower seed
- Sweet rice flour
- Tapioca
- Taro flour
- Teff
- Wild rice

Gluten-Free Additives (SAFE)

- Acacia gum (gum Arabic)
- Acetic acid
- Adipic acid
- Algin
- Annatto
- Aspartame
- Baking yeast
- Benzoic acid
- Beta carotene
- BHA
- BHT
- Brewer's yeast
- Brown sugar
- Calcium disodium EDTA
- Carrageenan
- Caramel color[1]
- Carboxymethyl cellulose
- Carob bean gum
- Cellulose
- Corn syrup

- Corn syrup solids
- Cream of tartar
- Dextrose
- Ethyl maltol
- Fructose
- Fumaric acid
- Gelatin
- Glucose
- Guar gum
- Invert sugar
- Karaya gum
- Lactic acid
- Lactose
- Lecithin
- Malic acid
- Maltodextrin[2]
- Maltol
- Mannitol
- Methlycellulose
- MSG—monosodium glutamate
- Papain
- Pectin
- Polysorbate 60; 80

- Propylene glycol
- Psyllium
- Sodium benzoate
- Sodium metabisulphite
- Sodium nitrate; Nitrite
- Sodium sulphite
- Sorbitol
- Stearic acid
- Sucralose
- Sucrose
- Sugar
- Tartaric acid
- Tartrazine
- Titanium dioxide
- Tragacanth
- Vanilla extract
- Vanillan
- White vinegar[3]
- Xanthan gum
- Xylitol
- Yam
- Yeast

[1] Caramel color is manufactured by heating carbohydrates and is produced from sweeteners. Although gluten-containing ingredients can be used, they are not used in North America; corn is most often used; however it is important to check with food manufacturers.

[2] Maltodextrin is made from cornstarch, potato starch, or rice starch.

[3] Distilled white vinegar is safe to consume on the gluten-free diet. Vinegar is a solution made of acetic acid and flavoring materials such as apples, grapes, grain, and molasses. For example, cider vinegar is made from apple juice; malt vinegar is made from barley malt, balsamic vinegar is made from grapes. Distilled vinegars are gluten-free because the distillation process filters out the large gluten proteins so that they do not pass through to the end product. Therefore, the finished liquid is gluten-free. Patients with celiac disease should not be concerned about distilled white vinegar or foods such as pickles, which may contain it. The exception to the rule is MALT VINEGAR, which is not distilled, and therefore is not safe to consume.

Here is a chart to help you determine which types of foods are safe and unsafe within various food groups. Again, it is highly recommended that a person newly diagnosed with celiac disease see an RD who specializes in treating people with celiac disease (and ideally diabetes, too).

Food Group or Type	AVOID
Grains and Beans	Products made from wheat, rye, barley, and regular oats
	Corn or rice cereals with added barley malt for flavor (i.e., regular corn flakes cereal)
	Items made with wheat bran, wheat farina, semolina, durum flour, kamut, matzo, panko bread crumbs, spelt, graham flour, or oatmeal
	Bulgur, couscous, orzo, tabbouleh
Soups	Canned soups containing gluten Bouillon cubes with gluten Canned broth with gluten

ALLOWED	CAUTION
Amaranth Arrowroot Beans (canned and dried): pinto, black, garbanzo, kidney, etc. Bean flours Buckwheat Cassava Corn Corn bran and corn flour Corn tortillas Cornmeal Cornstarch Flax Garbanzo, chickpea, lentil, or pea flour Lentils Millet Montina flour Nut flours Potatoes Potato starch, flour Quinoa Rice: white, brown, wild Sorghum Soy Tapioca (cassava flour) Teff Uncontaminated oats Yucca	Seasoned or flavored rice mixes or noodles may contain gluten. Some beans, such as "seasoned chili beans," may contain gluten. Read labels and check for gluten.
Gluten-free canned soups and broth Homemade broth and soups Gluten-free bouillon	Seasoned or flavored rice mixes or noodles may contain gluten. Some beans, such as "seasoned chili beans," may contain gluten. Read labels and check for gluten.

Food Group or Type	AVOID
Nuts and Seeds	Any seasoned nut or seed with gluten
Fruits	
Vegetables	Frozen vegetables with gluten-containing seasoning or sauce
	French fries (some frozen or those fried in contaminated fryer at restaurant)
	Breaded vegetables
Eggs	
Dairy	Cheese sauces, processed cheese, some ice cream
Meats	Lunch meats with gluten ingredients Breaded meats Imitation crabmeat Canned fish in gluten-containing broth Frozen turkey injected with gluten
Condiments and Vinegar	Soy sauce Malt vinegar
Fats	
Beverages	Malt-based drinks, such as Ovaltine Malted milk Malted milkshakes
Alcohol	Beer
	Some flavored alcohols, such as flavored vodkas and rum
	Wine coolers and bottled alcoholic beverages containing malt (includes wine coolers and some ciders)

ALLOWED	CAUTION
Plain nuts and seeds Naturally gluten-free nuts in the shell Nut flours	
Fresh, frozen, or canned fruit	
Fresh, frozen, canned plain vegetables without sauce	
Eggs	Read labels on egg products in carton.
Milk, most yogurt, and cheese	Read labels on yogurt, ice cream, and cheese to verify gluten-free ingredients. Avoid those with modified food starch, unspecified.
Lunch meats processed without gluten Fresh or frozen nonbreaded meats Most major brands of canned tuna	Read labels and check for gluten-containing ingredients in lunch meats, bacon, hot dogs, turkey, and canned tuna and salmon.
Gluten-free soy sauce Vinegar, except for malt vinegar	Read labels on all condiments and sauces to verify gluten-free ingredients. Barbeque and teriyaki sauce may contain gluten.
Butter, margarine, gluten-free salad dressing	Read labels on all salad dressing to verify gluten-free ingredients.
Coffee, tea, soda	Some teas can contain barley malt. Read ingredients and verify gluten-free status of all flavored coffees, teas, and specialty drinks.
Gluten-free beer Distilled alcohol, such as plain rum and vodka Wine	

CROSS-CONTAMINATION

Care must be taken in the kitchen to avoid cross-contamination. Even the tiniest amounts of gluten can cause a reaction in the short term; therefore, gluten must be completely avoided. Cross-contamination occurs when a gluten-free product comes in contact with one that contains gluten. Here are some tips to avoid cross-contamination:

- Gluten-free foods must be kept separate from gluten-containing foods. You may want to designate a separate cabinet or shelf in the pantry for gluten-free foods. A good tip is to store the gluten-free foods on a higher shelf than the gluten-containing foods.

- Purchase separate containers of foods, such as peanut butter, mayonnaise, and margarine, and label them as gluten-free. This eliminates contamination from the utensils used in gluten-containing products.

- Use separate cutting boards for gluten-free foods.

- Use a separate colander to drain gluten-free pasta.

- If you are using both gluten-free and gluten-containing foods, always prepare the gluten-free foods first. For example, if you are making a

Common Examples of Accidental Ingestion of Gluten
- Foods made with canned broth containing gluten (used to make sauces and rice at many restaurants)
- Foods fried in the same fryer with flour products: French fries at fast food restaurants and tortilla chips at Mexican restaurants
- Salad and fresh vegetables cut on the same cutting board as bread
- The same colander used to drain regular and gluten-free pasta
- Tea that contains malt
- Soy sauce that contains wheat used in marinade or other sauces
- Same spoon used to serve meat on flour and corn tortillas
- Breakfast meat, such as sausage or bacon, cooked on the same griddle or pan as regular pancakes
- Eating a hamburger that was simply taken off the bun
- Gluten-free pancakes cooked on the same grill as regular pancakes

gluten-free and a gluten-containing grilled cheese sandwich, always handle and prepare the gluten-free sandwich first.

- Make sure to wash your hands thoroughly between handling gluten-containing and gluten-free foods.

- Purchase a separate toaster for gluten-free bread because the crumbs from regular bread or waffles will contaminate the gluten-free product. If you use a toaster oven, line the grate with foil when preparing the gluten-free product.

- Make sure to thoroughly clean pots, pans, spoons, and countertops at all times.

- Be especially careful about cross-contamination when you eat out at restaurants or at someone's house.

EATING OUT

Research, care, and planning must be done when going out to eat with celiac disease. Many restaurants are now offering gluten-free menus or food items. Gluten-free restaurant information is available through many websites and phone apps.

Some Restaurants with Gluten-Free Menus or Options

- Biaggi's Ristorante Italiano
- Bonefish Grill
- Carraba's Italian Grill
- Cheeseburger in Paradise
- Cooper's Hawk Winery and Restaurant
- Flat Top Grill
- Francesca's Cucina
- Jason's Deli
- Legal Sea Foods
- Maggiano's Little Italy
- Melting Pot
- Mitchell's Fish Market
- Noodles and Company
- Outback Steakhouse
- PF Chang's Bistro
- Red Robin
- Stir-Crazy
- Ted's Montana Grill
- Weber Grill
- White Chocolate Grill
- Wildfire

Online Resources for Eating Out
- Allergy Eats (www.allergyeats.com)
- Find Me Gluten Free (www.findmeglutenfree.com)
- The Celiac Scene—Canada and U.S. (www.theceliacscene.com)
- Gluten-Free Allergy Free Passport (glutenfreepassport.com)
- Triumph Dining (www.triumphdining.com)
- Gluten-Free Restaurant Awareness Program (www.glutenfreerestaurants.org)

TRAVELING

Traveling with diabetes and celiac disease takes some investigating, planning, and packing. Just as people with diabetes need to remember to pack their glucose meter, test strips, medications, and/or insulin, you will need to investigate which restaurants offer gluten-free menus before you travel to your destination. You may want to plan to go to a local grocery store once you get to your destination. Almost all grocery stores offer some gluten-free options. If you are staying in a hotel, check to see if a refrigerator and microwave can be provided in your room. You will probably also want to pack some gluten-free foods and snacks while you are traveling.

Convenient Gluten-Free Foods for Traveling
- Individual peanut butter packs
- Gluten-free bread
- Gluten-free crackers
- Hot breakfast cereal (dry)—some instant gluten-free oatmeal packets are available
- Gluten-free bars, such as Kind Bars
- GoPicnic Ready to Eat Gluten-Free Meals
- Nuts
- Tuna pouches
- Enjoy Life Foods No Nuts Mountain Mambo Gluten-Free Trail Mix (snack pack size)
- Fruit

3

Diet Challenges and Recommendations for Diabetes and Celiac Disease

The double diagnosis of diabetes and celiac disease definitely has many challenges and can be overwhelming. Consider using these five steps for healthy gluten-free living.

FIVE STEPS FOR GLUTEN-FREE, DIABETES SURVIVAL

STEP 1: First and foremost the person with celiac disease must learn which foods are safe and which foods should be avoided. Make an appointment with an RD specializing in celiac disease. Ideally, this person will also be a certified diabetes educator (CDE) or have experience working with people who have diabetes as well.

STEP 2: While learning about gluten-free foods, try choosing fewer processed foods and more whole foods, such as sweet potatoes, fruit, vegetables, beans, legumes, fresh meat, and fish.

STEP 3: Take the proper steps to avoid cross-contamination in your kitchen.

STEP 4: If you can't tell if a product contains gluten, go to the company's website and see if you are able to find the information. If the information is not available on the website, call the company and ask if the product contains gluten. You can also try to email the company. If you are unable to reach the company and are still unsure, avoid the food.

STEP 5: Give yourself time to adjust to the new diet. It is normal to feel sad, overwhelmed, and angry about the fact that you have celiac disease. With time, you will get more accustomed to a gluten-free diet and learn how to live with it and still enjoy food. Focus on the foods you *CAN* eat. Check for local support groups, which can be a great way of meeting other people with celiac disease who can provide resources and recommendations. If you feel like you are not coping well, talk to you doctor and ask to be referred to a counselor or psychologist.

DIABETES AND CELIAC DISEASE DIET CHALLENGES

CHALLENGE #1
Many of the gluten-free substitutes for bread, rice, and crackers contain low-fiber, high-glycemic-index carbohydrates that may raise blood glucose levels.

SOLUTION #1
▶ Try to find the lowest-carbohydrate, highest-fiber gluten-free bread and crackers available. You can also eat corn tortillas or gluten-free, high-fiber wraps in place of bread. You can eat foods such as tuna salad and chicken salad with high-fiber gluten-free crackers. Look for baking, pancake, and flour blends with the highest fiber content or with a mix of flours that include some whole grains. For example, Bob's Red Mill All-Purpose Baking Flour is a blend of garbanzo bean flour, sorghum flour, tapioca flour, and fava bean flour. You can also add some gluten-free oats to your pancake or cookie batter to boost the fiber. Beans and legumes are a naturally high-fiber, gluten-free, healthy carbohydrate. Try to incorporate more beans into your diet by adding them to salads, soups, and taco meat, or by spreading hummus on your sandwich instead of mayonnaise. You can also purée beans or lentils and add them to meatloaf, brownies, or muffins.

CHALLENGE #2

The carbohydrate content of gluten-free foods can be higher than that of the traditional version. Most regular, gluten-containing bread contains about 15 grams of carbohydrate per slice, whereas one slice of gluten-free bread can range from 15 to 40 grams of carbohydrate per slice. Gluten-free hot dog buns range from 21 to 58 grams.

SOLUTION #2

▶ Read labels on every food item, and check the carbohydrate content, along with gluten-free status. Don't assume gluten-free products contain the same amount of carbohydrates as their gluten-containing counter-parts. Be sure to consider the total carbohydrate content as you manage your carbohydrate intake from day to day.

CHALLENGE #3

People may feel very restricted on a gluten-free diet and may want to binge or treat themselves to many gluten-free packaged foods all the time. Since the gluten-free food market has grown dramatically in the past couple years, it is very tempting to want to try every new gluten-free cookie, chip, bar, or brownie.

SOLUTION #3

▶ Try to restrain yourself. You don't have to worry about a shortage of delicious gluten-free foods because they are readily available now. You can treat yourself every now and then, but as with any meal plan, try to restrain from eating these high-fat, high-carbohydrate foods on a regular basis.

CHALLENGE #4

You may notice blood glucose levels are higher and are more difficult to control with the gluten-free diet.

SOLUTION #4

▶ A good way to see how different gluten-free foods are affecting your blood glucose is to test blood glucose levels two hours after meals. The American Diabetes Association recommends a target blood glucose of

180 mg/dl one to two hours after a meal. Make an appointment with an RD or CDE, so he or she can evaluate your food intake and glucose monitoring results. He or she can determine whether you can achieve your blood glucose goals by adjusting your foods and meals or if medication adjustments are needed.

CHALLENGE #5
Your diet is low in fiber and may be causing problems, such as constipation or feeling hungry all the time.

SOLUTION #5
▶ Include high-fiber, gluten-free foods in your diet every day. Foods that are high in fiber are whole grains, beans, fresh fruit, and vegetables. Also, see Solution #1.

CHALLENGE #6
You have gained weight with the start of the gluten-free diet.

SOLUTION #6
▶ Weight gain can happen when you start a gluten-free diet because when the intestines were in a damaged state, you were not absorbing many of the nutrients and calories that you were consuming. Therefore, you might have been able to eat more calories without gaining weight. As your intestines begin to heal, you may absorb more calories and experience weight gain. Weight gain can also occur because many of the gluten-free food products are higher in calories, carbohydrates, and fat than their counterparts.

WHAT ABOUT WHOLE GRAINS?

Many of the gluten-free substitutes for bread, pasta, crackers, and snacks are made of low-carbohydrate grains such as white rice. Although it isn't necessary to avoid these products entirely, it's healthier to choose whole-grain, gluten-free foods more often. Try various gluten-free whole grains (or products made from these grains) from this list:

Gluten-Free Whole Grains Include:

- Amaranth
- Buckwheat
- Millet
- Certified gluten-free oats
- Quinoa
- Sorghum
- Stone ground cornmeal
- Teff
- Wild rice

Examples of Gluten-Free Products that Contain Whole Grains:

- Gluten-free rolled oats
- La Tortilla Factory Gluten-Free Wraps
- Rudi's Gluten-Free Tortillas
- Crunchmaster Crackers
- Ancient Harvest Quinoa Flakes cereal
- Bob's Red Mill All-Purpose Baking Gluten-Free Flour
- Udi's Millet-Chia Bread
- Breads from Anna—Gluten-free bread and muffin mixes
- Orgran Buckwheat Pasta
- Ancient Harvest Quinoa Pasta

HIGH GLYCEMIC INDEX VERSUS LOW GLYCEMIC INDEX

As mentioned previously, many of the gluten-free commercial products can be made with high-glycemic-index (GI) starches, such as rice and potato flour. The GI of a food measures how quickly a carbohydrate-containing food raises blood glucose levels. Foods are ranked based on how they affect blood glucose levels compared with those of a reference food, either pure glucose or white bread. A food with a high GI raises blood glucose more than a food with a medium or low GI. Here are some examples of foods that rank higher versus lower on the GI scale.

Higher-Glycemic Index Gluten-Free Foods:

- White rice
- White potatoes
- Rice cakes and rice crackers
- Corn pasta
- Rice milk

Lower-Glycemic Index Gluten-Free Foods:

- Legumes and beans beans (e.g., garbanzo, black-eyed peas, kidney, black)
- Lentils
- Buckwheat
- Peas

Carbohydrate Content of Various Gluten-Free Products

Product	Serving Size	Carbohydrates (grams)	Fiber (grams)	Total Fat (grams)
Glutino Multigrain Bread	2 slices	20	<2	7
Udi's Whole Grain Bread	2 slices	22	1	4
Udi's Millet-Chia Bread	2 slices	24	5	4.5
Ancient Harvest Quinoa Pasta	2 ounces dry	46	4	1
Kettle Cuisine Turkey Chili with Beans	1 cup	22	7	4
Kinninick Blueberry Muffin	1 muffin	32	3	7
Mary's Gone Original Crackers	13 crackers	21	3	5
Crunchmaster Multi-grain Crackers	16 crackers	23	3	3
Beanito Black Bean Chips	1 ounce	5	5	7
Corn tortilla	1 tortilla (23.6g)	12	1	0
Kind Bar, almond coconut	1 bar	19	4	13
Rudi's Gluten-Free Plain Tortillas	1 tortilla (32g)	17	5	2.5
LaTortilla Factory Gluten-Free Wrap	1 wrap (66g)	30	3	5
Quinoa (cooked)	1/2 cup	20	2.6	2
Hot Buckwheat Cereal	1/4 cup dry	33	1	1

Always read labels to check carbohydrate content and verify gluten-free status.

- Sweet potato (baked)
- Quinoa
- Milk (1%, 2%, and fat-free milk)

Foods that contain very little carbohydrate and do not significantly raise blood glucose levels include:
- Low-carb vegetables, such as broccoli, cauliflower, green beans, asparagus, peppers, zucchini, Brussels sprouts, spinach, and many more.
- Protein foods, such as egg, fish, chicken, turkey, and beef, and pork.

GLUTEN-FREE DIET TIPS FOR PEOPLE WITH DIABETES

1. **Don't ever assume a food is gluten-free.** Don't say, "I'm sure this food can't have gluten in it." You will be surprised to find out that certain foods contain gluten. Regular corn flakes cereal, licorice, soy sauce, imitation crabmeat, many canned soups, and some flavored potato chips are just some examples of foods that contain gluten.

2. **Always read food labels.** People with diabetes are used to reading food labels and checking for carbohydrates. Make sure you continue to do this because many gluten-free products, such as bread, cereal, or cookies, may be higher in carbohydrates than their counterparts. You also want to verify gluten-free status by checking ingredients on the food label. If you are unsure if a food is gluten-free, check for information about the product on the company website or call the company. Many companies now have allergen information on their websites, and the gluten information can sometimes be found there.

3. **Call ahead and talk to the host about what they are serving when you are going to a dinner party.** You can always offer to bring a gluten-free, diabetes-friendly dish. Call ahead when attending a wedding or special event, too. Most banquet halls and large hotels are getting more accustomed to providing gluten-free meals at events.

4. **Choose healthy gluten-free carbohydrates more often.** If you had diabetes first, you were probably taught to choose healthy carbohydrates. Now this recommendation is the same but includes choosing healthy gluten-free carbohydrates.

Examples of Healthy Gluten-Free Carbohydrates

- Fresh fruit
- Nonfat or 1% milk
- Plain or light yogurt (verify gluten-free status)
- Beans, including garbanzo, black, pinto, Great Northern, kidney
- Lentils
- Whole-grain gluten-free bread
- Quinoa
- Wild rice
- Sweet potatoes
- Gluten-free rolled oats
- Crackers made with lentils or gluten-free whole grains
- Tortillas or wraps made with gluten-free whole grains

5. **Regularly check your blood glucose levels to see how your new diet affects your diabetes.** Because many gluten-free commercial products are low in fiber and higher in fat and carbohydrates, you may notice a change or elevation in your blood glucose levels if you are eating a lot of these foods. Postprandial blood glucose testing or testing two hours after a meal can give you information on how your blood glucose is responding to certain foods. The American Diabetes Association recommends blood glucose of 180 mg/dl or less two hours after a meal. Further, once you start a gluten-free diet, over time, your absorption of nutrients and oral medications improves, and this may require adjustments to your insulin and/or oral medications. An RD who is knowledgeable in celiac disease and diabetes can help you in this area, too.

6. **Don't assume just because a restaurant has a gluten-free menu that you are completely safe.** Make sure to ask questions about food preparation and menu items. Ask to talk to the manager or chef if you have questions.

7. **Keep your kitchen safe.** Purchase separate containers of foods that are at risk for cross-contamination, such as margarine tubs and jelly, peanut butter, and mayonnaise jars. You can label these containers as gluten-free with a permanent marker. Use a separate toaster and colander for

gluten-free bread and pasta to avoid cross-contamination. Make sure all of your pans, utensils, and cutting boards are clean and free from gluten before using. If you are preparing a regular meal and a gluten-free meal, always wash your hands after handling any gluten-containing foods.

8. **Get the family involved.** Your family needs to become familiar with gluten-free foods and what is safe for you to eat. It's important for your family to understand the importance of a strict gluten-free diet. As with diabetes, your spouse or other family members can go with you to your health-care appointments to learn as much as possible. There is a lot to learn, and often people have good intentions, but they lack the knowledge of how to safely prepare gluten-free food. Here are a few stories I've heard over the years on how family members accidentally fed gluten to people with celiac disease:

- Pot roast with potatoes and gluten-filled bouillon cube
- Serving packaged, cooked chicken that contained wheat
- Casseroles with rice and gluten-containing canned soups
- Salad dressing made with wheat-containing soy sauce
- Taking the croutons off of a salad and still serving it

CELIAC DISEASE, DIABETES, AND CHILDREN

More children with type 1 diabetes are being diagnosed with celiac disease today because doctors are screening them for celiac disease. Years ago, children with type 1 diabetes were not routinely screened for celiac disease, so there are probably many adults with type 1 diabetes who are not diagnosed with celiac disease.

Parents and children may have finally gotten used to dealing with checking blood glucose levels, taking insulin injections, counting carbohydrates, and then . . . a celiac disease diagnosis. It just doesn't seem fair. So, now in addition to all these changes, children with this double diagnosis must follow a gluten-free diet.

Here's the good news—children are amazing and seem to adapt to things better than we often expect. I've seen some patients who've had diabetes for 50 or more years and their diligence and compliance in avoiding sugar and following a regimented lifestyle always inspire me. Insulin and diet recommendations for diabetes were very different 50 years ago. These patients were told to eat three meals per day at the same time every day and avoid sugar or sweet treats, and many of them still do this same regimen 50 years later. They will tell you that this is all they knew as a child and that it was easy to continue this lifestyle as an adult.

The gluten-free diet can be very healthy for both kids and adults (with or without diabetes). Gluten-free eating forces people to eat less fast food and when done correctly, it can include more natural foods such as fruits, vegetables, beans, and healthy protein. Here are some tips for helping children adapt to gluten-free eating:

- Always try to provide a gluten-free alternative to any food served at a school event or party. Sometimes you might find that the other kids prefer the gluten-free food option, too. You could also encourage schools to offer only fruit and vegetable snacks. These are naturally gluten-free and better for growing bodies.

- Just as kids are involved in learning about diabetes, they should also learn to identify what foods contain gluten and what foods are gluten-free. This comes with time for all of us; just make sure to include your child in this learning process.

- Talk positively about the gluten-free diet. Your child will hear you, and their opinion will be more positive.

- Make gluten-free eating tasty and fun! This rule can apply to all kids— make it fun and tasty and they are more likely to eat healthy foods. Try making a "Green Smoothie" with baby spinach, a banana, milk, and some yogurt. Your kids will love this healthy treat. Kids love to dip things, so serve veggies and gluten-free hummus or apple slices with peanut butter on the side to dip.

- Have kids help in preparing meals and snacks. Kids love to create things, and they will be more interested in eating something that they've helped make. Try making gluten-free pumpkin or zucchini muffins since kids love to break eggs and mixing things.

Check out the Resource Section at the end of the book for other tools for children with celiac disease.

4

Putting It All Together
Gluten-Free, Diabetes-Friendly Meal Planning

THE HEALTHY PLATE

Try to keep healthy eating simple by using the Healthy Plate as a guide and modify the plate to include gluten free foods.

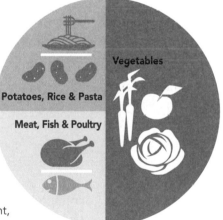

1. **FILL 1/2 OF THE PLATE WITH LOW-CARB VEGGIES:**
   Examples: green beans, broccoli, cauliflower, salad, spinach, zucchini, eggplant, asparagus, greens, or tomatoes

2. **FILL 1/4 OF THE PLATE WITH HEALTHY, GLUTEN-FREE CARBOHYDRATES:**
   Examples: beans, legumes, quinoa, sweet potatoes, multigrain gluten-free bread, or crackers

3. **FILL 1/4 OF THE PLATE WITH PROTEIN:**
   Examples: chicken breast, turkey, fish, lean pork, lean beef, or eggs

CARB COUNTING

Carbohydrate (carb) counting is a meal planning approach used by people with diabetes to assist in blood glucose control.

Basic Carb Counting

Basic carb counting is tracking the amount of carbohydrates eaten at meals and snacks. A person is given a target number of carbohydrates to eat at meals and snacks in order to manage blood glucose levels and maintain weight or aid in weight loss (if needed). By reading food labels and using resources to look up the carbohydrate content of certain foods, people can determine how much carbohydrate they are eating. All packaged gluten-free foods will come with a food label, and reading food labels is an essential part of carb counting. An RD or CDE can work with you to help you with carb counting.

An RD or CDE should determine how much carbohydrate you should eat at each meal. The following is a general guideline, but carbohydrate recommendations for adults will also vary based on your health status, exercise, age, and need for weight loss or maintenance.

ADULT WOMEN: 30–45 grams carbohydrate per meal

ADULT MEN: 60–75 grams carbohydrate per meal

SNACKS FOR ADULTS: 15–20 grams per snack

CHILDREN—carbohydrate recommendations will vary based on age and activity level.

Advanced Carb Counting

Advanced carb counting allows people to match their dose of rapid-acting insulin to the amount of carbohydrate they eat. Exercise and blood glucose levels before the meal are also taken into account for calculating the dose of rapid-acting insulin. This can lead to improved blood glucose control because people receive their insulin in a fashion similar to they way it is released by a healthy pancreas. An insulin-to-carbohydrate ratio is the amount of carbohydrate that is "covered" by 1 unit of rapid-acting insulin. Your ratio may vary for each meal and may change with weight gain or loss or based on exercise.

An RD or CDE can work with you to assist in determining and adjusting these ratios if needed.

5

Gluten-Free, Diabetes-Friendly
Grocery Lists, Menus, and Snacks

GLUTEN-FREE HEALTHY GROCERY LIST

CARBOHYDRATES

Starchy Foods
- Gluten-free multigrain bread (choose highest fiber content available)
- Gluten-free wraps
- Corn tortillas
- Brown or wild rice
- Quinoa
- Cereal with 3 or more grams dietary fiber, e.g., Nature's Path Whole O's
  or Barbara's Gluten-Free Puffins
- Oats (gluten-free)
- Gluten-free crackers, e.g., Mary's Gone and Crunchmaster
- Sweet potatoes
- Dried or canned beans, e.g., pinto, kidney, red, refried beans
- Gluten-free bars, e.g., Kind Bars, BumbleBar, or NuGo
- Gluten-free waffles
- Beanito Chips or Food Should Taste Good Multigrain Chips

Fruits
- Fresh fruit
- Canned fruit in juice

Milk and Yogurt
- 1% or nonfat (skim) milk
- Almond milk
- Light yogurt or Greek yogurt

Desserts
- Light or low-fat ice cream
- Sugar-free pudding, gelatin dessert, and frozen pops

Miscellaneous
- Glutino frozen dinners
- GoPicnic Ready-to-Eat Gluten-Free Meals
- Gluten-free soups—choose bean and lentil more often
- Gluten-free all-purpose flour with fiber, e.g., Bob's Red Mill

NONCARBOHYDRATES

Meat and Meat Substitutes
- Skinless chicken breast
- Lean ground turkey
- Lean beef and pork, round or loin cuts, e.g., sirloin, tenderloin
- Fish
- Canned tuna, packed in water (verify that it is gluten-free)
- Gluten-free lunch meats, e.g., Hormel Natural Choice turkey breast, ham, lean beef
- Light cheese
- Low-fat or fat-free cottage cheese
- Eggs

Vegetables
- Fresh or frozen vegetables

Fats
- Light cream cheese
- Light sour cream
- Light salad dressings
- Light mayonnaise or Miracle Whip
- Olive or canola oil
- Tub margarine, e.g., Smart Balance
- Cooking spray
- Peanuts, almonds, nuts

- Avocado and olives
- Peanut butter

Beverages
- Flavored calorie-free waters
- Crystal Light and diet soda

Miscellaneous
- Gluten-free chicken broth, e.g., Pacific brand

Always verify gluten-free status on all products. Higher fiber choices are listed here when available. This list is not inclusive. There are many brands and options for healthy gluten-free foods. The ADA does not endorse any gluten-free product or company.

GLUTEN-FREE MENUS

Gluten-Free Breakfasts with 30 Grams Total Carbohydrate or Less

BREAKFAST #1

1 slice gluten-free bread, served with 1 teaspoon sugar-free jam

1 hard-boiled egg

1 cup strawberries

BREAKFAST #2

1/2 cup low-fat cottage cheese

1/2 cup pineapple

1 slice gluten-free bread, served with 1 teaspoon trans-fat-free margarine

BREAKFAST #3

6 ounces plain, fat-free Greek yogurt

1 1/2 cups blueberries

1 tablespoon sliced almonds

BREAKFAST #4

1 corn tortilla

1 egg OR 1/4 cup egg substitute

(add 1 ounce reduced-fat cheese and veggies, such as green pepper and
   onion, to eggs when cooking)

1 cup mixed berries

*Combine ingredients in the tortilla to make a burrito served with berries on
   the side.*

BREAKFAST #5

1 cup unsweetened almond milk

1 cup unsweetened frozen berries

2 ounces plain, fat-free Greek yogurt

Put in a blender and mix for a delicious smoothie.

BREAKFAST #6

1/2 cup egg substitute

1 cup chopped spinach (or vegetables of your choice)

1/2 cup diced tomato

2 tablespoons reduced-fat cheddar cheese

1 slice gluten-free bread, toasted

1 slice Canadian bacon

Prepare omelet with first four ingredients, serve with toast and Canadian bacon.

Gluten-Free Breakfasts with 45 Grams Total Carbohydrate

BREAKFAST #1

1 egg OR 1/4 cup egg substitute, cooked with

1 ounce low-sodium ham, served on

    2 slices gluten-free bread (to lower carbohydrates, serve on corn tortillas instead)

1 cup melon

Serve as a sandwich with melon on the side.

BREAKFAST #2

1/2 cup gluten-free hot cereal (aim for 4 grams fiber per serving), served with cinnamon

1 tablespoon chopped walnuts

1 cup fat-free milk

BREAKFAST #3

1 gluten-free waffle, served with

    2 teaspoons peanut butter

4 ounces plain, fat-free Greek yogurt

1 cup strawberries

Gluten-Free Lunches with 30 Grams Total Carbohydrate or Less

LUNCH #1 (CHICKEN WRAP)

1 gluten-free tortilla

3 ounces chicken

1/8 avocado, mashed (spread on tortilla)

1/4 cup diced tomatoes

Serve chicken, avocado, and tomatoes wrapped in the tortilla.

LUNCH #2

Large green salad, with

    3 ounces cooked chicken breast

    1 tablespoon chopped pecans

    2 tablespoons balsamic vinaigrette dressing (gluten-free)

1 cup gluten-free black bean soup

LUNCH #3 (CHICKEN SALAD)

3 ounces cooked chicken, chopped, mixed with

    1 tablespoon light mayo

    chopped onion

    1/4 cup grapes, halved

    1 tablespoon slivered almonds

10 gluten-free crackers

1/2 cup cottage cheese

1/2 cup strawberries

Serve chicken salad on gluten-free crackers with strawberries and cottage
cheese on the side.

LUNCH #4 (EGG WHITE SALAD)

3 hard-boiled egg whites, mixed with

    1 tablespoon light mayo

    1 teaspoon Dijon mustard, served on

Mixed greens OR 14 multigrain tortilla chips

1 cup fresh fruit

Gluten-Free Lunches with 45 Grams Total Carbohydrate

LUNCH #1 (TURKEY OR HAM WRAP)

1 gluten-free tortilla, filled with
    3 ounces low-sodium ham or turkey
    1 tablespoon hummus
    lettuce leaves
    tomato slices
1 small apple
Small green salad, with
    1 tablespoon light dressing (gluten-free)

LUNCH #2 (TUNA SALAD)

3 ounces water-packed tuna, with
    1 tablespoon light mayo
    chopped celery
    chopped onion, served on
    2 slices gluten-free bread
1 cup carrots, cucumbers, and cauliflower, served with
    2 tablespoons hummus
1 cup milk or 6 ounces light yogurt
Serve tuna salad on bread with veggies, hummus, and yogurt on the side.

LUNCH #3

1 cup gluten-free canned soup (lentil or black bean)
1/2 natural peanut butter and sunflower seed sandwich, made with
    1 slice gluten-free bread
    1 tablespoon peanut butter
    2 teaspoons sunflower seeds
1 cup strawberries

LUNCH #4

3 ounces leftover chicken breast, chopped, mixed with
    1/2 cup fat-free refried beans, served on
    14 multigrain tortilla chips OR two corn tortillas
Green salad, with
    2 tablespoons light ranch dressing (gluten-free)
1 medium orange

Gluten-Free Dinners with 30 Grams Total Carbohydrate

DINNER #1

Chicken stir-fry made with

    3–4 ounces chicken breast (season with gluten-free soy sauce and spices)

1 cup stir-fried vegetables

2/3 cup wild rice

DINNER #2

Lean hamburger served on

    2 slices gluten-free multigrain bread

1 cup green beans

Sugar-free gelatin dessert

DINNER #3

Grilled pork chop

1/2 cup mashed cauliflower

1/2 cup broccoli

1/2 cup light ice cream, served with

    3/4 cup strawberries

DINNER #4

Chopped chicken salad, made with

    3 cups chopped romaine lettuce

    3–4 ounces chicken breast, chopped

    1/2 cup black beans

    1/8 avocado, sliced

    1/2 hard-boiled egg

    2 tablespoons reduced-fat dressing

1 cup melon

Mix chicken salad ingredients in a bowl and toss to coat.

Gluten-Free Dinners with 45 Grams Total Carbohydrate

DINNER #1

1 baked sweet potato, served with

    1 tablespoon trans-fat-free margarine

3 ounces grilled pork tenderloin

1 cup cooked broccoli

DINNER #2
3–4-ounce salmon fillet
2/3 cup cooked quinoa pilaf
6–7 asparagus spears
3/4 cup berries

DINNER #3
Turkey tacos, made with
    3–4 ounces ground turkey
    2 corn tortillas
    1/2 cup black beans
    lettuce
    tomato
    reduced-fat cheese
1 cup melon

DINNER #4
1 cup chili with beans
1 small corn muffin
Large green salad, with
    1 tablespoon reduced-fat dressing

LOW-CARB SNACKS

Here are some examples of snacks with 15–20 grams of carbohydrate:
- 8–10 whole-grain gluten-free crackers with 1 tablespoon peanut butter
- 1 small pear and a small handful (12) almonds
- 4 ounces flavored Greek yogurt
- 3 cups popcorn
- 1/2 cup sugar-free pudding
- 1/2 cup peaches and 1/2 cup low-fat cottage cheese
- 1 small protein or nut bar with around 15 grams carbohydrate
- 1 small apple with 1 tablespoon peanut butter
- 4 baby carrots, 4 celery stalks dipped in 2 tablespoons hummus
- 1 corn tortilla with 1 slice turkey and 1 tablespoon reduced-fat shredded cheese, heated in the microwave

Here are some examples of snacks with less than 15 grams of carbohydrate:

- Small handful of almonds, walnuts, or pecans
- 3 celery stalks with 1 tablespoon peanut butter
- String cheese
- Light cheese wedge spread on cucumber slices
- 1/2 cup low-fat cottage cheese
- Hard-boiled egg
- Sugar-free gelatin dessert with 1 tablespoon light whipped topping

Some of these menus and snacks were adapted from *Healthy Calendar Diabetic Cooking, 2nd edition* (American Diabetes Association 2012).

GLUTEN-FREE
RECIPES

APPETIZERS/SNACKS

Practice Gluten Awareness
Be sure to always verify that your ingredients are gluten-free. Products do
change over time; so don't assume that since a product was safe before,
it will always be gluten-free.

AVOCADO-TOMATILLO SALSA

Serves 8 • Serving Size: 1/4 cup • Makes 2 cups salsa total

---

  1 ripe medium avocado, peeled, seeded, and chopped
1/2 cup diced tomatoes
1/4 cup diced green bell pepper OR 1 medium jalapeño, seeded
     and finely chopped
1/4 cup diced red onion
  1 medium tomatillo, papery skin removed and diced (about 2 ounces)
1/4 cup chopped cilantro
  2 tablespoons lemon juice
  1 teaspoon cider vinegar
1/4 teaspoon salt

---

1. In a medium bowl, combine all ingredients.

COOK'S TIP	Take a break from the corn tortillas and serve with raw veggies, such as cucumber, jicama, bell peppers, or on Belgian endive.

EXCHANGES/FOOD CHOICES		
1 Vegetable, 1/2 Fat	Cholesterol	0 mg
	Sodium	75 mg
	Potassium	160 mg
BASIC NUTRITIONAL VALUES:	Total Carbohydrate	3 g
Calories	40	Dietary Fiber	2 g
Calories from Fat	25	Sugars	1 g
Total Fat	3.0 g	Protein	1 g
Saturated Fat	0.4 g	Phosphorus	20 mg
Trans Fat	0.0 g		

LAYERED-UP BEAN DIP

Serves 12 • Serving Size: 1/3 cup • Makes 4 cups

---

  1 16-ounce can fat-free refried beans
  1 4-ounce can diced mild green chilies
  1 cup diced tomato
1/2 cup finely chopped green onion
1/2 cup chopped cilantro
1/2 cup fat-free sour cream (read labels)
1/2 teaspoon ground cumin
  1 ounce shredded reduced-fat sharp cheddar cheese (1/4 cup)
  1 medium avocado, pitted, peeled, and diced
  1 medium lime, cut in half

---

1. Spread the refried beans in the bottom of a 9-inch pie pan. Sprinkle chilies, tomato, green onion, and cilantro evenly over all.
2. In a small bowl, stir together sour cream and cumin. Place sour cream, by small spoonfuls, over the top. Sprinkle evenly with the cheese and avocado. Squeeze lime juice over all.

COOK'S TIP Many times, layered bean dips are made with taco seasoning mixes that contain gluten.

EXCHANGES/FOOD CHOICES
1/2 Carbohydrate, 1/2 Fat

BASIC NUTRITIONAL VALUES:

Calories	75	Cholesterol	0	mg
Calories from Fat	20	Sodium	220	mg
Total Fat	2.5 g	Potassium	280	mg
Saturated Fat	0.6 g	Total Carbohydrate	10	g
Trans Fat	0.0 g	Dietary Fiber	3	g
		Sugars	1	g
		Protein	4	g
		Phosphorus	80	mg

SPANISH OLIVE AND HERBED HUMMUS

Serves 8 • Serving Size: 3 tablespoons • Makes 1 1/2 cups

1	15-ounce can no-salt-added Great Northern or navy beans, rinsed and drained
1/2	cup nonfat plain Greek yogurt
12	small stuffed green olives
1–2	medium garlic cloves, peeled only
1 1/2	tablespoons extra-virgin olive oil
1	tablespoon lemon juice
1	tablespoon water
1/2	teaspoon dried oregano leaves
1/4	teaspoon dried rosemary
1/4	teaspoon salt
1/8	teaspoon dried pepper flakes, optional

---

1. Combine all ingredients in a blender, until smooth.

COOK'S TIP Serve with raw veggies or rice tortilla wedges.

EXCHANGES/FOOD CHOICES
1/2 Starch, 1/2 Fat

BASIC NUTRITIONAL VALUES:

Calories	80	Cholesterol	0 mg
Calories from Fat	30	Sodium	160 mg
Total Fat	3.5 g	Potassium	155 mg
Saturated Fat	0.5 g	Total Carbohydrate	8 g
Trans Fat	0.0 g	Dietary Fiber	3 g
		Sugars	1 g
		Protein	4 g
		Phosphorus	75 mg

CROSTINI WITH GREEN PEPPER-KALAMATA RELISH

Serves 4 • Serving Size: 4 bread pieces and 1/4 cup tomato mixture •
Makes 16 bread pieces and 1 cup tomato mixture

Base
    4   slices gluten-free whole-grain bread, such as Udi's, cut into 4 squares each
    2   medium garlic cloves, peeled and halved crosswise

Topping
    1/2   cup finely chopped tomato
     8   pitted kalamata olives, diced
    1/4   cup diced green bell pepper OR 1 medium jalapeño, seeded and
          minced
     2   tablespoons diced red onion
     2   tablespoons chopped fresh basil
     1   tablespoon cider vinegar

---

1. Arrange the bread squares on a baking sheet. Place in the oven and set the
   oven for 350°F. Do NOT preheat oven. Bake for 5 minutes on each side.
   Cool completely.

2. Meanwhile, in a small bowl, combine the topping ingredients.

3. Rub the tops of the bread with the garlic and serve topped with the tomato
   mixture.

EXCHANGES/FOOD CHOICES			
1 Starch, 1/2 Fat		Cholesterol	0 mg
		Sodium	215 mg
		Potassium	240 mg
BASIC NUTRITIONAL VALUES:		Total Carbohydrate	14 g
Calories	95	Dietary Fiber	2 g
Calories from Fat	35	Sugars	3 g
Total Fat	4.0 g	Protein	3 g
Saturated Fat	0.2 g	Phosphorus	60 mg
Trans Fat	0.0 g		

HOUSE-MADE CORN TORTILLA CHIPS

Serves 8 • Serving Size: 6 chips • Makes 48 chips

---

8 6-inch soft corn tortillas (read labels)

4 teaspoons canola oil

Seasoning

1 1/2 teaspoons chili powder

3/4 teaspoon ground cumin

1/2 teaspoon garlic powder

1/4 teaspoon onion powder

1/2 teaspoon salt

---

1. Preheat oven to 350°F.
2. Brush each tortilla lightly with 1/2 teaspoon oil. Stack and cut into 6 sections, making 48 wedges. Arrange in a single layer on two large cookie sheets.
3. In a small bowl, combine the remaining ingredients, except the salt. Sprinkle evenly over all and bake 11–12 minutes or until lightly golden. Remove from heat, sprinkle evenly with the salt, and cool completely on cookie sheet.
4. When cooled, store in airtight containers up to 2 weeks for peak texture and flavor.

COOK'S TIP	This is a great recipe to serve alone or with your favorite salsa or dip.

EXCHANGES/FOOD CHOICES		Cholesterol	0 mg
1 Starch, 1/2 Fat		Sodium	155 mg
		Potassium	50 mg
BASIC NUTRITIONAL VALUES:		Total Carbohydrate	12 g
Calories	75	Dietary Fiber	1 g
Calories from Fat	25	Sugars	0 g
Total Fat	3.0 g	Protein	1 g
Saturated Fat	0.3 g	Phosphorus	80 mg
Trans Fat	0.0 g		

SMOKY, CRUNCHY SNACK MIX

Serves 10 • Serving Size: 1/2 cup • Makes 5 cups

---

  1 tablespoon gluten-free Worcestershire sauce
  1 tablespoon prepared mustard
  1 tablespoon canola oil
  4 cups gluten-free Corn or Rice Chex-style cereal
  2 ounces gluten-free pretzels, broken into bite-size pieces
  2 ounces hulled pumpkin seeds, salted
  2 teaspoons smoked paprika
  1 teaspoon ground cumin
1/2 teaspoon garlic powder
1/8 teaspoon cayenne, optional
1/4 teaspoon salt

---

1. Preheat the oven to 300°F.
2. In a small bowl, stir together the Worcestershire sauce, mustard, and oil. Combine the cereal, pretzels, and pumpkin seeds in a large bowl. Drizzle the Worcestershire sauce mixture over all and toss gently, yet thoroughly, until well coated. Sprinkle evenly with the paprika, cumin, garlic powder, and cayenne. Toss gently until well blended.
3. Place the cereal mixture on a large nonstick cookie sheet in a thin layer. Bake 8 minutes, stir, and bake 7 minutes or until golden.
4. Remove from oven, place on wire rack, and cool completely on cookie sheet. Sprinkle evenly with the salt.
5. Store in an airtight container in dry storage up to 2 weeks for peak flavors and texture.

| COOK'S TIP | Store in 1/2 cup batches in sandwich baggies for individual servings. |

EXCHANGES/FOOD CHOICES
1 Starch, 1 Fat

BASIC NUTRITIONAL VALUES:

Calories	115
Calories from Fat	45
Total Fat	5.0 g
Saturated Fat	0.7 g
Trans Fat	0.0 g
Cholesterol	0 mg
Sodium	265 mg
Potassium	120 mg
Total Carbohydrate	16 g
Dietary Fiber	1 g
Sugars	1 g
Protein	3 g
Phosphorus	85 mg

PEPPERONI POTATO HALVES

Serves 8 • Serving Size: 3 halves • Makes 24 halves

KID FRIENDLY

12	new potatoes (about 1 1/4 pounds total), pierced with a fork in several areas
16	slices turkey pepperoni, finely chopped
1 1/2	ounces grated part-skim mozzarella cheese
2	tablespoons freshly grated Parmesan cheese
1	tablespoon canola oil
2	tablespoons finely chopped roasted red peppers
2	teaspoons dried basil leaves
1/8	teaspoon dried pepper flakes, optional

1. Place potatoes on a microwave-safe plate, cover, and cook on high setting 10 minutes or until tender when pierced with a fork.

2. Meanwhile, combine the remaining ingredients in a small bowl, fluff with a fork.

3. Remove potatoes from microwave and let stand 10 minutes for easier handling. Cut potatoes in half lengthwise, place potato halves, cut side up, on 2 microwave-safe dinner plates, spoon equal amounts of the pepperoni mixture on each potato half. Working with one plate at a time, microwave on high for 1–2 minutes or until cheese is melted slightly. Let stand 3 minutes before serving. Serve warm.

EXCHANGES/FOOD CHOICES		Cholesterol	10 mg
1 Starch, 1/2 Fat		Sodium	135 mg
		Potassium	280 mg
BASIC NUTRITIONAL VALUES:		Total Carbohydrate	14 g
Calories	100	Dietary Fiber	1 g
Calories from Fat	30	Sugars	1 g
Total Fat	3.5 g	Protein	4 g
Saturated Fat	1.0 g	Phosphorus	115 mg
Trans Fat	0.0 g		

FREEZER-TO-OVEN MINI MOZZARELLA STICKS

Serves 6 • Serving Size: 3 sticks • Makes 18 mini cheese sticks

KID FRIENDLY

6	reduced-fat mozzarella cheese sticks, such as Weight Watchers, cut in thirds crosswise
1	tablespoon gluten-free all-purpose flour
1/4	cup low-fat buttermilk
1/2	cup gluten-free bread crumbs, such as Gillian's
1 1/2	teaspoons dried oregano leaves
1/4	teaspoon garlic powder
1/4	teaspoon paprika
	Cooking spray
1	8-ounce can no-salt-added tomato sauce or Italian tomato sauce, optional

1. Place the cheese stick pieces in a shallow pan, such as a pie pan, sprinkle with the flour, and toss to coat. Pour the buttermilk in a small bowl. Combine the breadcrumbs, oregano, garlic powder, and paprika in another shallow pan, such as a pie pan.

2. Working with one at a time, dip cheese stick pieces into the buttermilk and coat with the breadcrumb mixture. Place in a single layer on a large plate. Freeze until firm.

3. Preheat oven to 400°F.

4. Coat a foil-lined baking sheet with cooking spray. Arrange the frozen cheese stick pieces in a single layer, being careful not to touch each other. Bake 5 minutes, turn, and bake 4–5 minutes or until crisp, being careful not to melt.

5. Serve as is or with tomato sauce for dipping.

EXCHANGES/FOOD CHOICES		Cholesterol	5 mg
1 Med-Fat Meat		Sodium	160 mg
		Potassium	45 mg
BASIC NUTRITIONAL VALUES:		Total Carbohydrate	3 g
Calories	65	Dietary Fiber	0 g
Calories from Fat	20	Sugars	0 g
Total Fat	2.5 g	Protein	7 g
Saturated Fat	1.1 g	Phosphorus	140 mg
Trans Fat	0.0 g		

APPLES WITH NUTTY CARAMEL FRUIT DIP

Serves 4 • Serving Size: 1/4 piece (1/2 cup apple slices and 2 tablespoons sauce) • Makes 2 cups apple slices and 1/2 cup sauce

KID FRIENDLY

1/4 cup gluten-free, reduced-fat peanut butter
1/4 cup sugar-free caramel ice cream topping
2 tablespoons fat-free milk
2 medium apples, thinly sliced

1. Place peanut butter in a small microwave-safe bowl. Microwave on high setting for 30 seconds. Remove from microwave and whisk in the ice cream topping. Whisk in the milk. Serve with apple slices.

EXCHANGES/FOOD CHOICES		
1/2 Fruit, 1 1/2 Carbohydrate, 1 Fat	Cholesterol	0 mg
	Sodium	95 mg
	Potassium	200 mg
BASIC NUTRITIONAL VALUES:	Total Carbohydrate	27 g
Calories	175	Dietary Fiber	2 g
Calories from Fat	55	Sugars	8 g
Total Fat	6.0 g	Protein	4 g
Saturated Fat	1.0 g	Phosphorus	90 mg
Trans Fat	0.0 g		

THREE-CEREAL COOKIE MOUNDS

Serves 12 • Serving Size: 1 cookie • Makes 12 cookies

KID FRIENDLY

2	ounces slivered almonds or coarsely crushed peanuts
2	ounces hulled salted pumpkin seeds
1 1/2	cups gluten-free rice cereal
1	cup gluten-free corn flakes
1/2	cup gluten-free rolled oats
1/8	teaspoon ground cinnamon
1/4	teaspoon salt
2	cups miniature marshmallows OR 4 ounces marshmallow cream
2	tablespoons canola oil

1. Place a large saucepan over medium-high heat until hot, add nuts and pumpkin seeds, cook 2–3 minutes or until fragrant and beginning to lightly brown, stirring constantly.

2. Place in a medium bowl, add rice cereal, corn cereal, oats, cinnamon, and salt, toss gently, yet thoroughly, to blend.

3. Place the large saucepan over medium heat, add marshmallows and oil, stir until completely melted. Remove from heat, add cereal mixture; using a rubber spatula, stir constantly about 1 minute or until melted and beginning to stick together.

4. Working quickly, spoon equal amounts into a 12-cup muffin tin and shape slightly. Cool completely.

EXCHANGES/FOOD CHOICES			
1 Carbohydrate, 1 1/2 Fat		Cholesterol	0 mg
		Sodium	115 mg
		Potassium	90 mg
BASIC NUTRITIONAL VALUES:		Total Carbohydrate	16 g
Calories	140	Dietary Fiber	1 g
Calories from Fat	65	Sugars	6 g
Total Fat	7.0 g	Protein	3 g
Saturated Fat	0.8 g	Phosphorus	105 mg
Trans Fat	0.0 g		

BREAKFAST

Practice Gluten Awareness
Be sure to always verify that your ingredients are gluten-free. Products do change over time; so don't assume that since a product was safe before, it will always be gluten-free.

NUTTY CRANBERRY-OAT GRANOLA

Serves 18 • Serving Size: 1/3 cup • Makes 6 cups granola mixture

KID FRIENDLY

---

4 cups gluten-free rolled oats
2 ounces sliced almonds
2 ounces chopped pecans
2 ounces hulled sunflower seeds
1/4 teaspoon plus 1/4 teaspoon salt, divided
1/4 cup honey
1/4 cup packed Splenda Brown Sugar Blend
1 tablespoon canola oil
1 tablespoon water
2 teaspoons vanilla
1/2 cup dried cranberries
1 tablespoon grated lemon rind

---

1. Preheat the oven to 300°F. Coat a baking sheet with cooking spray.

2. In a large bowl, combine the oats, almonds, pecans, sunflower seeds, and 1/4 teaspoon salt. Add the honey, Splenda Brown Sugar Blend, oil, water, and vanilla, stirring constantly. Spread on the baking sheet about 1/4 inch thick. Bake for 30 minutes or until browned.

3. Remove from the oven, stir, and sprinkle evenly with the remaining 1/4 teaspoon salt, cranberries, and lemon rind. Do not stir. Cool completely on baking sheet. Store in an airtight container in the refrigerator for up to 2 weeks.

EXCHANGES/FOOD CHOICES		
1 Starch, 1/2 Carbohydrate, 1 1/2 Fat	Cholesterol	0 mg
	Sodium	65 mg
	Potassium	145 mg
BASIC NUTRITIONAL VALUES:	Total Carbohydrate	25 g
Calories	185	Dietary Fiber	3 g
Calories from Fat	70	Sugars	8 g
Total Fat	8.0 g	Protein	5 g
Saturated Fat	0.8 g	Phosphorus	160 mg
Trans Fat	0.0 g		

PINEAPPLE-MANGO PARFAITS

Serves 4 • Serving Size: 1/2 cup yogurt, 1/3 cup cereal mixture,
1/4 cup mango, and 1/4 cup pineapple • Makes 4 parfaits

KID FRIENDLY

---

2 cups gluten-free Rice Chex-style cereal, coarsely crushed
1 ounce slivered almonds, coarsely crushed
2 tablespoons packed Splenda Brown Sugar Blend
2 cups plain nonfat Greek yogurt
1 ripe medium mango, peeled, pitted, and cut into 1/2-inch cubes
1 8-ounce can pineapple tidbits in their own juice, drained

---

1. In a small bowl combine cereal, almonds, and Splenda Brown Sugar Blend.

2. In four dessert bowls or parfait glasses, spoon equal amounts of the yogurt in each. Top with equal amounts of the cereal mixture, mango, and pineapple.

EXCHANGES/FOOD CHOICES		
1 Starch, 1 Fruit, 1 Fat-Free Milk	Cholesterol	0 mg
	Sodium	160 mg
	Potassium	340 mg
BASIC NUTRITIONAL VALUES:	Total Carbohydrate	39 g
Calories	245	Dietary Fiber	2 g
Calories from Fat	35	Sugars	23 g
Total Fat	4.0 g	Protein	14 g
Saturated Fat	0.4 g	Phosphorus	205 mg
Trans Fat	0.0 g		

OK OATMEAL WITH STRAWBERRIES AND ALMONDS

Serves 4 • Serving Size: 1/2 cup oatmeal and 1/2 cup topping •
Makes 2 cups oatmeal and 2 cups topping

- 1 cup gluten-free rolled oats
- 2 cups water
- 1/4 teaspoon salt
- 1/4 cup raspberry fruit spread, slightly melted
- 1/2 teaspoon almond extract
- 2 cups strawberries, quartered
- 1 ounce slivered almonds, toasted

---

1. Combine water, oats, and salt in a medium-size pan. Bring to a boil, reduce heat, and simmer 10 minutes uncovered. Remove from heat, let stand 2 minutes.

2. Place the fruit spread in a small microwave-safe bowl and cook on high setting for 15 seconds or until slightly melted. Remove from heat, stir in the extract.

3. Spoon equal amounts of the oatmeal in 4 bowls. Top with 1 tablespoon fruit spread, 1/2 cup berries, and 1 tablespoon almonds.

EXCHANGES/FOOD CHOICES			
1 Starch, 1 Fruit, 1 Fat			
		Cholesterol	0 mg
		Sodium	160 mg
		Potassium	265 mg
BASIC NUTRITIONAL VALUES:		Total Carbohydrate	33 g
Calories	205	Dietary Fiber	5 g
Calories from Fat	55	Sugars	12 g
Total Fat	6.0 g	Protein	5 g
Saturated Fat	0.6 g	Phosphorus	170 mg
Trans Fat	0.0 g		

PEACHES AND SWEET CREAMED HOT QUINOA CEREAL

Serves 4 • Serving Size: 1/2 cup cereal, 1/4 cup cream, and 1/3 cup peach mixture • Makes 2 cups cereal, 1 cup cream, and 1 1/3 cups peach mixture

---

Topping
- 1 cup diced peaches or mango
- 1/3 cup dried cranberries (optional)
- 1 tablespoon packed Splenda Brown Sugar Blend

Cereal
- 2 cups water
- 2/3 cup quinoa flakes, such as Ancient Harvest
- 1/4 teaspoon salt
- 1 tablespoon packed Splenda Brown Sugar Blend

Cream
- 1 cup fat-free half-and-half
- 1 tablespoon packed Splenda Brown Sugar Blend
- 1 teaspoon vanilla

---

1. In a small bowl, combine the peaches, cranberries, and 1 tablespoon of the Splenda Brown Sugar Blend.
2. In a large saucepan, bring the water to boil over high heat. Stir in quinoa flakes and salt. Boil for 1 1/2 minutes, stirring frequently. Remove from heat, stir in the remaining tablespoon sugar substitute. Let stand, covered, 3 minutes to thicken slightly.
3. Place the half-and-half in a small microwave-safe bowl and heat in microwave on high for 2 minutes or until heated. Stir in 1 tablespoon of the sugar substitute and the vanilla.
4. Spoon equal amounts of the quinoa in four cereal bowls, pour the half-and-half mixture evenly over all, and spoon equal amounts of the peach mixture on top of each.

COOK'S TIP Quinoa flakes is a hot cereal that is different than the grain. It is sold in health-food stores and major supermarkets.

EXCHANGES/FOOD CHOICES
1 Starch, 1/2 Fat-Free Milk,
    1 Carbohydrate

BASIC NUTRITIONAL VALUES:

Calories	190
Calories from Fat	20
Total Fat	2.5 g
Saturated Fat	0.6 g
Trans Fat	0.0 g
Cholesterol	5 mg
Sodium	210 mg
Potassium	360 mg
Total Carbohydrate	37 g
Dietary Fiber	2 g
Sugars	12 g
Protein	5 g
Phosphorus	215 mg

DOWN HOME HASH BROWN SKILLET

Serves 4 • Serving Size: 1 1/4 cups • Makes 5 cups

1	tablespoon canola oil, divided
4	ounces diced extra-lean ham
1 1/2	cups diced onion
2	poblano chile peppers, seeded and diced OR 1 cup diced green bell pepper
1	pound red or Yukon gold potatoes, scrubbed and diced
1/2	teaspoon dried thyme leaves
1/2	teaspoon black pepper
1/8	teaspoon cayenne, optional
1 1/2	ounces shredded reduced-fat sharp cheddar cheese
1	cup grape tomatoes, quartered

---

1. Heat 1 teaspoon of the oil in large nonstick skillet; brown ham over medium heat, about 2 minutes. Set aside on separate plate.

2. Heat 1 teaspoon of the oil, cook the onions and peppers 4 minutes or until lightly browned. Heat the remaining 1 teaspoon oil and stir in the potatoes, thyme, black pepper, and cayenne. Cook, uncovered, for 14 minutes, or until potatoes are tender, stirring occasionally.

3. Remove from the heat, stir in the ham, top with the cheese and tomatoes. Cover and let stand 5 minutes for peak flavor and texture of the potatoes.

EXCHANGES/FOOD CHOICES
1 Starch, 2 Vegetable, 1 Lean Meat, 1 Fat

BASIC NUTRITIONAL VALUES:

Calories	230	Trans Fat	0.0 g
Calories from Fat	70	Cholesterol	20 mg
Total Fat	8.0 g	Sodium	440 mg
Saturated Fat	2.2 g	Potassium	835 mg
		Total Carbohydrate	29 g
		Dietary Fiber	4 g
		Sugars	6 g
		Protein	12 g
		Phosphorus	220 mg

ENGLISH MUFFIN BREAKFAST STACKS

Serves 4 • Serving Size: 1 stack • Makes 4 stacks

---

2 gluten-free English muffins, cut in half to make 4 rounds total
1 tablespoon gluten-free light mayonnaise
1 tablespoon nonfat yogurt
2 Canadian bacon slices (2 ounces total)
1 2.5-ounce container diced pimiento OR 1/4 cup diced tomato
1 ounce shredded reduced-fat sharp cheddar cheese

---

1. Preheat broiler. Place muffin halves on a cookie sheet and broil 1–2 minutes on each side until lightly toasted.

2. In a small bowl stir together the mayonnaise and yogurt, and spread mixture evenly over the muffins. Top with bacon slices and equal amounts of pimiento and cheese. Broil 2–3 minutes or until bubbly.

EXCHANGES/FOOD CHOICES		
1 1/2 Starch, 1 Lean Meat, 1/2 Fat		

Cholesterol	15	mg
Sodium	470	mg
Potassium	250	mg

BASIC NUTRITIONAL VALUES:		
Calories	180	
Calories from Fat	45	
Total Fat	5.0	g
Saturated Fat	1.4	g
Trans Fat	0.0	g

Total Carbohydrate	22	g
Dietary Fiber	1	g
Sugars	4	g
Protein	7	g
Phosphorus	115	mg

FRENCH TOAST WITH LEMON-BERRY TOPPING

Serves 4 • Serving Size: 1 French toast slice, 1 tablespoon sauce,
2 tablespoons yogurt, and 2 tablespoons berries • Makes 4 French toast
slices, 1/4 cup sauce, 1/2 cup yogurt, and 1/2 cup berries

Toast

- 2 teaspoons canola oil
- 1/2 cup gluten-free egg substitute
- 1/4 cup fat-free milk
- 1 teaspoon vanilla
- 4 gluten-free bread slices, such as Udi's Millet-Chia variety

Topping

- 2 1/2 tablespoons raspberry fruit spread
- 1 1/2 tablespoons water
- 1/2 teaspoon grated lemon rind
- 1/2 cup plain nonfat Greek yogurt
- 1/2 cup blueberries

1. Heat the oil in a large nonstick skillet over medium heat.

2. Stir together the egg substitute, milk, and vanilla in a 13-inch by 9-inch baking pan, add bread slices, and turn several times to coat evenly. Cook the bread slices 3 minutes on each side or until golden.

3. Meanwhile, place the fruit spread and water in a small microwave-safe bowl and microwave on high for 15 seconds to melt slightly. Stir in the lemon rind.

4. Place toast slices on each of four plates, spoon fruit spread mixture over all, and top with the yogurt and berries.

EXCHANGES/FOOD CHOICES		
1 Starch, 1/2 Carbohydrate, 1 Lean Meat, 1/2 Fat		
	Trans Fat	0.0 g
	Cholesterol	0 mg
	Sodium	220 mg
	Potassium	205 mg
BASIC NUTRITIONAL VALUES:	Total Carbohydrate	23 g
Calories	170	
	Dietary Fiber	3 g
Calories from Fat	40	
	Sugars	11 g
Total Fat	4.5 g	
	Protein	10 g
Saturated Fat	0.3 g	
	Phosphorus	160 mg

EGG AND GREEN CHILE TORTILLA MELTS

Serves 4 • Serving Size: 1 sandwich (1 cup egg mixture and 1 tortilla) • Makes 4 cups egg mixture and 4 tortillas

---

4	slices turkey bacon
1 1/2	cups gluten-free egg substitute, such as Egg Beaters
4	6-inch soft corn tortillas (read labels)
1	4-ounce can mild chopped green chilies
1	ounce shredded part-skim mozzarella cheese

---

1. Cook the bacon in a large nonstick skillet over medium heat. Drain bacon on paper towels. Crumble and set aside. Discard bacon grease.
2. Return the skillet to medium heat. Add the eggs. Cook 1 minute, do not stir. Then, gently lift to allow uncooked egg to flow under. When cooked, remove skillet from heat. Spoon the green chilies on top of the eggs, sprinkle evenly with the cheese and bacon. Place over medium-low heat, cover, and cook 2 minutes to heat through.
3. Meanwhile, warm tortillas in microwave according to package directions. Spoon equal amounts of the egg mixture on top of each tortilla.

EXCHANGES/FOOD CHOICES
1 Starch, 2 Lean Meat

BASIC NUTRITIONAL VALUES:

Calories	155	Cholesterol	10 mg
Calories from Fat	35	Sodium	470 mg
Total Fat	4.0 g	Potassium	255 mg
Saturated Fat	1.5 g	Total Carbohydrate	15 g
Trans Fat	0.0 g	Dietary Fiber	2 g
		Sugars	1 g
		Protein	14 g
		Phosphorus	160 mg

HEARTY BANANA MUFFINS WITH PINEAPPLE TOPPING

Serves 12 • Serving Size: 1 muffin • Makes 12 muffins

Muffins
        Cooking spray
1 1/4 cups gluten-free, all-purpose baking flour, such as Bob's Red Mill
1 1/2 teaspoons baking powder
2 1/2 teaspoons ground cinnamon
  1/4 teaspoon salt
  3/4 cup low-fat buttermilk
  1/2 cup gluten-free egg substitute OR 4 egg whites
  1/4 cup packed Splenda Brown Sugar Blend
    2 tablespoons canola oil
    1 teaspoon vanilla, butter, and nut flavoring OR 2 teaspoons vanilla extract
    1 cup mashed ripe bananas

Topping
    2 8-ounce cans pineapple tidbits in their own juice, drained
    1 tablespoon sugar
  1/4 teaspoon ground cinnamon

1. Preheat oven to 350°F. Lightly spray muffin tin with cooking spray, set aside.

2. In a medium bowl, whisk together the flour, baking powder, 2 1/2 teaspoons cinnamon, and salt. In another medium bowl, whisk together the remaining muffin ingredients, except the bananas, until just blended. Stir in the bananas.

3. Spoon into prepared muffin tins. Top with equal amounts of the pineapple. Bake 22 minutes or until wooden pick inserted comes out clean and the muffins are slightly brown on the edges. Let stand in tins 15 minutes before removing.

4. In a small bowl, combine the sugar and remaining 1/4 teaspoon cinnamon. Sprinkle evenly over all.

EXCHANGES/FOOD CHOICES
1 1/2 Carbohydrate, 1/2 Fat

BASIC NUTRITIONAL VALUES:

Calories	130
Calories from Fat	25
Total Fat	3.0 g
Saturated Fat	0.3 g
Trans Fat	0.0 g

Cholesterol	0 mg
Sodium	130 mg
Potassium	200 mg
Total Carbohydrate	24 g
Dietary Fiber	2 g
Sugars	10 g
Protein	3 g
Phosphorus	105 mg

APPLE-PECAN PUMPKIN COFFEE CAKES

Serves 16 • Serving Size: 1 wedge (1/8 cake) • Makes two 9-inch coffee cakes

---

Cakes

    Cooking spray
1 15-ounce box gluten-free yellow cake mix
1/4 cup canola oil
2/3 cup water
3/4 cup egg substitute OR 6 large egg whites
1 cup solid pumpkin
1 1/2 teaspoons vanilla extract or vanilla, butter, and nut flavoring
2 teaspoons ground cinnamon
1/4 teaspoon ground nutmeg

Topping

4 cups diced apples (about 4 medium Jonathan or Gala apples)
1/2 teaspoon ground nutmeg
4 ounces chopped pecans
1/4 cup packed Splenda Brown Sugar Blend

---

1. Preheat oven to 325°F. Coat bottom only of two nonstick 9-inch round (or square) cake pans with cooking spray.

2. In a large bowl, combine the cake ingredients and prepare according to package directions. Spoon batter into the pans and top with the apples; sprinkle 1/2 teaspoon nutmeg and pecans evenly over all.

3. Bake for 25 minutes or until wooden pick inserted comes out clean. Place pan on cooling rack, sprinkle evenly with the Splenda Brown Sugar Blend, and cool completely. Cut into wedges.

EXCHANGES/FOOD CHOICES		Cholesterol	0 mg
2 Carbohydrate, 2 Fat		Sodium	165 mg
		Potassium	195 mg
BASIC NUTRITIONAL VALUES:		Total Carbohydrate	33 g
Calories	215	Dietary Fiber	2 g
Calories from Fat	80	Sugars	16 g
Total Fat	9.0 g	Protein	3 g
Saturated Fat	0.8 g	Phosphorus	55 mg
Trans Fat	0.0 g		

PEACH-PEAR FRUIT SPREAD

Serves 32 • Serving Size: 1 tablespoon • Makes 2 cups

---

12   ounces frozen unsweetened peach slices, thawed and diced
 1   large firm pear, peeled, halved, cored, and diced
1/4 cup raisins or dried cherries
1/2 cup water
 1   tablespoon cornstarch
1/2 teaspoon ground cinnamon
 1   tablespoon trans-fat-free margarine
 2   tablespoons pourable sugar substitute
 1   teaspoon vanilla extract

---

1. Combine the peaches, pears, raisins, 2 tablespoons of the water, cornstarch, and cinnamon in a medium saucepan. Stir until cornstarch is dissolved. Bring to boil over medium-high heat. Boil 1 minute, stirring frequently. Reduce heat, cover, and simmer 7–9 minutes or until pears are just tender.
2. Remove from heat, stir in the margarine, and cool completely in the pan. When cooled, stir in the sugar substitute and vanilla. Refrigerate leftovers in an airtight container up to 2 weeks.

Note: The fruit will continue to cook while cooling down in the pan.

EXCHANGES/FOOD CHOICES
Free food

BASIC NUTRITIONAL VALUES:
Calories   15
  Calories from Fat 0
Total Fat   0.0 g
  Saturated Fat   0.0 g
  Trans Fat   0.0 g

Cholesterol   0 mg
Sodium   0 mg
Potassium   35 mg
Total Carbohydrate 3 g
  Dietary Fiber   0 g
  Sugars   2 g
Protein   0 g
Phosphorus   0 mg

SANDWICHES

Practice Gluten Awareness

Be sure to always verify that your ingredients are gluten-free. Products do change over time; so don't assume that since a product was safe before, it will always be gluten-free.

LAZY CHICKEN QUESADILLAS

Serves 2 • Serving Size: 2 quesadillas • Makes 4 quesadillas (4 tortillas,
1 1/3 cups mixture, and 1/2 cup topping)

KID FRIENDLY

1/2 cup gluten-free picante sauce
1/2 cup diced cooked chicken breast
1 ounce shredded part-skim mozzarella
1/4 teaspoon ground cumin
1 teaspoon canola oil
Cooking spray
4 6-inch soft corn tortillas (read labels)
1/4 cup diced tomatoes
1/4 cup fat-free sour cream (read labels)

1. Place the picante sauce in a fine mesh sieve and drain well, discarding about
1 tablespoon of the liquid. Combine the chicken, picante sauce, cheese,
and cumin in a medium bowl, toss lightly until well blended.

2. Heat oil in a large nonstick skillet over medium heat. Lightly coat one side of
each tortilla with cooking spray and place sprayed side down in skillet.
Spoon equal amounts of the mixture on top of each tortilla (about 1/3 cup
each) Using a fork, lightly spread chicken mixture evenly over each tortilla.
Cook 2 minutes, fold over, and press down with a fork to adhere. Then cook
2 minutes on each side or until golden and cheese has melted.

3. Top each quesadilla with 1 tablespoon diced tomatoes and 1 tablespoon
sour cream.

COOK'S TIP You can double this recipe. Keep the first 4 quesadillas warm in a preheated 200°F oven while preparing the remaining 4 quesadillas.

EXCHANGES/FOOD CHOICES
1 1/2 Starch, 1/2 Carbohydrate,
2 Lean Meat, 1/2 Fat

BASIC NUTRITIONAL VALUES:

Calories	275	Trans Fat	0.0 g
Calories from Fat	70	Cholesterol	40 mg
Total Fat	8.0 g	Sodium	595 mg
Saturated Fat	2.3 g	Potassium	415 mg
		Total Carbohydrate	32 g
		Dietary Fiber	4 g
		Sugars	3 g
		Protein	19 g
		Phosphorus	345 mg

PIECE O' PIZZA

Serves 4 • Serving Size: 1/2 individual pizza • Makes 2 pizzas

KID FRIENDLY

2	frozen gluten-free pizza crusts (8 ounces total)
1/2	cup no-salt-added tomato sauce
1	ounce pine nuts, toasted
1/2	cup chopped fresh basil leaves
1	teaspoon chopped fresh rosemary
1/4	teaspoon dried red pepper flakes
16	slices (1 ounce) turkey pepperoni
6	ounces sliced mushrooms
1/2	cup (2 ounces) thinly sliced red onion
1	cup thinly sliced green bell pepper
3/4	ounce shredded part-skim mozzarella
2	teaspoons freshly grated Parmesan cheese

1. Preheat oven to 375°F.
2. Place the pizza rounds on large cookie sheet. Spread equal amounts of tomato sauce on each. Sprinkle equal amounts of the remaining ingredients, except the cheeses, in the order listed.
3. Bake 12 minutes or until crust is golden on edges. Remove from oven, turn on broiler. Sprinkle mozzarella evenly over all and broil 45 seconds to melt cheese. Remove from broiler and sprinkle with Parmesan cheese. Cut into wedges.

EXCHANGES/FOOD CHOICES			Trans Fat	0.0 g
2 Starch, 1 Vegetable, 1 Lean Meat, 2 Fat			Cholesterol	20 mg
			Sodium	595 mg
			Potassium	720 mg
BASIC NUTRITIONAL VALUES:			Total Carbohydrate	39 g
Calories		320	Dietary Fiber	4 g
Calories from Fat		115	Sugars	9 g
Total Fat		13.0 g	Protein	13 g
Saturated Fat		2.4 g	Phosphorus	350 mg

GRILL PAN SAUSAGE DOGS

Serves 4 • Serving Size: 1 sandwich (1 sausage dog plus about 2 teaspoons
sauce and 1/3 cup vegetables) • Makes 4 sandwiches

    Cooking spray
 1 medium red onion, cut in 1/2-inch thick slices
 1 medium green bell pepper, cut in fourths lengthwise, seeds and stem
    discarded
 2 Italian chicken sausage links, such as Al Fresco sweet Italian style with
    red and green peppers, cut in half lengthwise
 4 gluten-free hot dog buns

Sauce
     2 teaspoons gluten-free light mayonnaise
2 1/2 tablespoons plain nonfat yogurt
   1/2 teaspoon Splenda Brown Sugar Blend
   1/2 teaspoon prepared mustard
   1/8 teaspoon ground cinnamon
   1/8 teaspoon cayenne

---

1. Lightly coat a grill pan with cooking spray and place over medium-high
   heat. Lightly coat onions and peppers with cooking spray and place on
   grill pan with sausage. Cook 12 minutes, stirring occasionally.
2. Meanwhile, in a small bowl stir together the sauce ingredients. Set aside.
3. Place sausage and vegetables on cutting board and coarsely chop the
   vegetables. Lightly coat the buns with cooking spray, grill 30 seconds on
   each side watching closely not to burn.
4. To assemble, place sausage link halves on top of buns. Spoon equal
   amounts of the sauce and vegetables on top.

EXCHANGES/FOOD CHOICES		Trans Fat	0.0 g
2 Starch, 1 Vegetable, 1 Lean Meat, 1 Fat		Cholesterol	35 mg
		Sodium	595 mg
		Potassium	620 mg
BASIC NUTRITIONAL VALUES:		Total Carbohydrate	37 g
Calories	280	Dietary Fiber	5 g
Calories from Fat	90	Sugars	7 g
Total Fat	10.0 g	Protein	13 g
Saturated Fat	1.6 g	Phosphorus	230 mg

TORTILLA TOPPERS

Serves 4 • Serving Size: 2 tortillas (6 tablespoons bean spread and
1/2 cup topping) • Makes 8 tortillas

Bean Spread

    1   15-ounce can no-salt-added black beans, rinsed and drained
1/4 cup chopped cilantro
1/4 cup diced red onion
    2 tablespoons lime juice
    2 tablespoons water
1/4 teaspoon ground cumin
1/4 teaspoon salt
1/4 teaspoon cayenne

Salsa

1 1/2 cups diced tomatoes
  1/4 cup diced red onion
   16 pitted ripe olives, coarsely chopped
  1/4 cup chopped cilantro
  1/4 teaspoon salt

    8 6-inch soft corn tortillas (read labels)
    1 ripe medium avocado, peeled and seeded
 1/2 cup fat-free sour cream (read labels)
    1 medium lime, quartered

---

1. Combine the bean spread ingredients in a blender. Purée until smooth.
2. Combine the salsa ingredients in a medium bowl and set aside.
3. Warm tortillas according to package directions. Spread 3 tablespoons of
   the bean spread on top of each tortilla; top with equal amounts of salsa,
   avocado, and sour cream. Serve with lime wedges.

EXCHANGES/FOOD CHOICES
2 1/2 Starch, 2 Vegetable, 1 1/2 Fat

BASIC NUTRITIONAL VALUES:

Calories	320
Calories from Fat	80
Total Fat	9.0 g
Saturated Fat	1.4 g
Trans Fat	0.0 g
Cholesterol	5 mg
Sodium	455 mg
Potassium	805 mg
Total Carbohydrate	54 g
Dietary Fiber	10 g
Sugars	6 g
Protein	11 g
Phosphorus	330 mg

MEDITERRANEAN CHEESE GRILLERS

Serves 4 • Serving Size: 1 sandwich • Makes 4 sandwiches

Spread
- 2 ounces shredded part-skim mozzarella cheese
- 12 pitted kalamata olives, finely chopped
- 2 medium garlic cloves, minced
- 1 1/2 teaspoons chopped fresh oregano OR 1/2 teaspoon dried oregano

Filling
- 8 slices gluten-free multigrain bread
- 4 teaspoons Dijon mustard
- 12 large basil leaves
- 2 medium tomatoes (about 6 1/2 ounces each as purchased) cut into 4 slices each
- 1 tablespoon canola oil

1. In a small bowl, combine the spread ingredients and set aside.
2. Place four bread slices on a clean work surface. Top each bread slice with equal amounts of the cheese mixture, 3 basil leaves, and 2 tomato slices. Spread one side of the remaining bread slices with the mustard and place mustard side down on top of the tomatoes.
3. Heat the oil in a large nonstick skillet over medium heat. Place the sandwiches in the skillet and cook 2–3 minutes on each side, or until golden.

EXCHANGES/FOOD CHOICES
1 1/2 Starch, 1 Vegetable, 2 1/2 Fat

BASIC NUTRITIONAL VALUES:

Calories	250
Calories from Fat	115
Total Fat	13.0 g
Saturated Fat	2.0 g
Trans Fat	0.0 g
Cholesterol	10 mg
Sodium	600 mg
Potassium	540 mg
Total Carbohydrate	28 g
Dietary Fiber	4 g
Sugars	6 g
Protein	9 g
Phosphorus	185 mg

SWEET AND SLOPPY SLIDERS

Serves 6 • Serving Size: 1 sandwich (1/2 cup beef mixture and 1 bun) •
Makes 3 cups beef mixture

KID FRIENDLY

12	ounces extra-lean (93% lean) ground beef
1 1/2	cups frozen mixed vegetables
7	tablespoons gluten-free medium picante sauce
1 1/2	tablespoons no-salt-added tomato paste
1 1/2	teaspoons cider vinegar
2	teaspoons packed Splenda Brown Sugar Blend
6	gluten-free hamburger buns, lightly toasted

1. Heat a large nonstick skillet over medium-high heat. Brown the beef, stirring frequently. Stir in the remaining ingredients, except the hamburger buns. Bring to a boil over medium-high heat, reduce heat, cover, and simmer 10 minutes or until vegetables are tender.
2. Spoon equal amounts on each of the hamburger buns.

EXCHANGES/FOOD CHOICES		
2 1/2 Starch, 1 Vegetable,	Trans Fat	0.2 g
1 Lean Meat, 1 1/2 Fat	Cholesterol	35 mg
	Sodium	585 mg
	Potassium	765 mg
BASIC NUTRITIONAL VALUES:	Total Carbohydrate	43 g
Calories 330	Dietary Fiber	6 g
Calories from Fat 90	Sugars	6 g
Total Fat 10.0 g	Protein	17 g
Saturated Fat 2.1 g	Phosphorus	260 mg

HEARTY SOUPS AND STEWS

Practice Gluten Awareness
Be sure to always verify that your ingredients are gluten-free. Products do change over time; so don't assume that since a product was safe before, it will always be gluten-free.

ON THE HEALTHY RUN
CHICKEN-CILANTRO SOUP

Serves 4 • Serving Size: 1 1/2 cups • Makes 6 cups

---

  2 cups frozen corn kernels
  1 15-ounce can no-salt-added black beans, rinsed and drained
  1 14.5-ounce can no-salt-added stewed tomatoes
  1 4-ounce can chopped mild green chilies
  1 14-ounce can reduced-sodium, gluten-free chicken broth
     (or bouillon and water)
  1 cup cooked chopped chicken breast meat
1/2 cup chopped cilantro
  1 tablespoon extra-virgin olive oil
1/4 teaspoon salt
  1 medium lime, quartered

---

1. In a large saucepan, combine the corn, beans, tomatoes, chilies, broth, and chicken. Bring to a boil, reduce heat, cover, and simmer 5 minutes.
2. Remove from heat, stir in the cilantro, oil, and salt. Serve with lime wedges.

COOK'S TIP   This is especially flavorful using leftover grilled chicken.

EXCHANGES/FOOD CHOICES
2 Starch, 1 Vegetable, 2 Lean Meat

BASIC NUTRITIONAL VALUES:

Calories	275	Cholesterol	30 mg
Calories from Fat	55	Sodium	535 mg
Total Fat	6.0 g	Potassium	925 mg
Saturated Fat	1.0 g	Total Carbohydrate	40 g
Trans Fat	0.0 g	Dietary Fiber	8 g
		Sugars	10 g
		Protein	20 g
		Phosphorus	280 mg

COUNTRY ROAD CHICKEN NOODLE SOUP

Serves 4 • Serving Size: 1 1/2 cups • Makes 6 cups

2	teaspoons canola oil, divided
3	boneless chicken breasts, trimmed of fat (12 ounces total)
1	cup diced onion
2	medium garlic cloves, minced
3	cups water
2	ounces dried corn pasta, such as elbow
1	cup thinly sliced carrots
1	cup diced red bell pepper
1/2	cup thinly sliced celery
3	packets gluten-free, sodium-free chicken bouillon granules
3/4	teaspoon dried thyme leaves
2	dried bay leaves
3	tablespoons gluten-free, trans-fat-free margarine
3/4	teaspoon salt

---

1. Heat 1 teaspoon of the oil in a large saucepan over medium heat. Cook the chicken 4 minutes on each side or until slightly pink in center. Place on cutting board and set aside.

2. Heat the remaining teaspoon oil in the saucepan. Cook the onions for 3 minutes or until translucent, stirring frequently. Add the garlic and cook 15 seconds, stirring constantly. Add the water; bring to a boil over high heat. Stir the pasta, carrots, bell peppers, celery, bouillon, thyme, and bay leaves into the onion mixture in saucepan. Return to a boil. Reduce the heat and simmer covered 15 minutes or until celery is tender.

3. Meanwhile, cut the chicken into bite-size pieces. Remove saucepan from heat, stir in chicken, margarine, and salt. Cover and let stand 5 minutes to absorb flavors.

COOK'S TIP	The chicken will continue to cook without drying out while resting on cutting board.

EXCHANGES/FOOD CHOICES
1 Starch, 1 Vegetable, 2 Lean Meat,
    1 Fat

BASIC NUTRITIONAL VALUES:

Calories	255
Calories from Fat	80
Total Fat	9.0 g
Saturated Fat	1.9 g
Trans Fat	0.0 g
Cholesterol	50 mg
Sodium	585 mg
Potassium	845 mg
Total Carbohydrate	23 g
Dietary Fiber	4 g
Sugars	6 g
Protein	21 g
Phosphorus	235 mg

SMOKED SAUSAGE-POTATO BEAN SOUP

Serves 8 • Serving Size: 1 cup • Makes 8 cups

1	tablespoon plus 1 teaspoon extra-virgin olive oil, divided
14	ounces gluten-free lean smoked turkey sausage, diced
1 1/2	cups diced onion
2	medium green bell peppers, seeded and chopped
3	medium carrots, thinly sliced
12	ounces red potatoes, diced
1	15-ounce can no-salt-added Great Northern beans, rinsed and drained
1/4	teaspoon dried pepper flakes
1	cup reduced-sodium, gluten-free chicken broth
2	cups water
1/4	cup chopped fresh parsley

---

1. Heat 1 teaspoon of the oil in a Dutch oven over medium-high heat. Brown sausage, about 4–5 minutes, stirring occasionally. Set aside on separate plate. Add the onions, peppers, carrots, potatoes, beans, and pepper flakes. Bring to a boil over high heat, reduce heat, cover, and simmer 20 minutes or until potatoes are tender.

2. Remove from heat. Stir in the sausage, parsley, and remaining 1 tablespoon oil. Using a potato masher or handheld blender, briefly mash or purée to thicken soup slightly. Cover and let stand 20 minutes to absorb flavors. This soup is even better the next day.

COOK'S TIP	Use the blender or potato masher to thicken a soup naturally . . . there's no need for flour or cornstarch! Or add gluten-free instant mashed potatoes for a double-quick and creamy soup! Or mash some of the beans before adding them. The mashing not only provides thickening without adding other ingredients, such as flours or cornstarch, but it allows the flavors to permeate the soup . . . in every bite.

EXCHANGES/FOOD CHOICES
1 Starch, 1 Vegetable, 1 Lean Meat,
  1 Fat

BASIC NUTRITIONAL VALUES:

Calories	215
Calories from Fat	65
Total Fat	7.0 g
Saturated Fat	1.7 g
Trans Fat	0.0 g
Cholesterol	25 mg
Sodium	585 mg
Potassium	620 mg
Total Carbohydrate	25 g
Dietary Fiber	5 g
Sugars	5 g
Protein	12 g
Phosphorus	220 mg

WHITE BEAN-RED PEPPER CHILI

Serves 4 • Serving Size: 1 1/4 cups (1 tablespoon sour cream and
1 tablespoon cilantro) • Makes 5 cups

2	tablespoons extra-virgin olive oil, divided
1	cup diced onion
1	cup diced red bell pepper
1	14.5-ounce can fat-free, reduced-sodium chicken broth
1	cup water
1 1/2	cups cooked diced chicken breast meat
1	16-ounce can no-salt-added navy beans, rinsed and drained
2	4.5-ounce cans chopped green chilies
2	teaspoons ground cumin
1/4	cup fat-free sour cream (read labels)
1/4	cup chopped cilantro

---

1. Heat 1 tablespoon of the oil in a Dutch oven over medium-high heat.
   Cook the onions and peppers 4 minutes or until just beginning to brown
   on edges, stirring frequently. Stir in the broth, water, chicken, beans, green
   chilies, and cumin. Bring to a boil over high heat. Reduce heat, cover, and
   simmer 10 minutes.

2. Remove from heat. Using a potato masher mash the chili mixture to thicken
   slightly. Stir in the remaining oil. Serve topped with sour cream and cilantro.

EXCHANGES/FOOD CHOICES		
1 Starch, 2 Vegetable, 3 Lean Meat, 1 Fat	Trans Fat	0.0 g
	Cholesterol	45 mg
	Sodium	475 mg
	Potassium	670 mg
BASIC NUTRITIONAL VALUES:	Total Carbohydrate	32 g
Calories 315	Dietary Fiber	9 g
Calories from Fat 90	Sugars	5 g
Total Fat 10.0 g	Protein	26 g
Saturated Fat 1.6 g	Phosphorus	290 mg

CHIPOTLE CREAMY TOMATO SOUP

Serves 4 • Serving Size: 1 1/4 cups • Makes 5 cups

1 1/2 tablespoons extra-virgin olive oil, divided
1 1/2 cups diced onion
   2 14.5-ounce cans no-salt-added diced tomatoes
1/2 15-ounce can no-salt-added navy beans, rinsed and drained
   1 medium chipotle chile pepper
   2 teaspoons adobo sauce (from canned chipotle chilies)
   2 ounces light cream cheese, tub style, cut into small pieces
1/2 teaspoon salt
   1 cup fat-free half-and-half
1/2 cup fat-free sour cream (read labels)

1. Heat 1 teaspoon of the oil in a large saucepan. Cook onion until beginning to lightly brown, about 4 minutes, stirring frequently. Stir in the tomatoes, beans, chipotle pepper, and the sauce. Bring to a boil over high heat, reduce heat, cover, and simmer 25 minutes or until onions are very tender; remove from heat.
2. Working in batches, purée the tomato mixture in a blender (be sure to hold down lid). Return to the saucepan. Whisk in the half-and-half and cream cheese. Place over medium heat and cook until heated through and cheese has melted. Remove from heat, stir in the salt and remaining 2 teaspoons oil. Serve topped with sour cream.

EXCHANGES/FOOD CHOICES
1/2 Starch, 1 Fat-Free Milk,
2 Vegetable, 1 1/2 Fat

BASIC NUTRITIONAL VALUES:

Calories	260	Trans Fat	0.0 g	
Calories from Fat	100	Cholesterol	15 mg	
Total Fat	11.0 g	Sodium	565 mg	
Saturated Fat	3.1 g	Potassium	745 mg	
		Total Carbohydrate	35 g	
		Dietary Fiber	7 g	
		Sugars	13 g	
		Protein	9 g	
		Phosphorus	245 mg	

HOME-STYLE BURGUNDY BEEF STEW

Serves 4 • Serving Size: 1 1/4 cups • Makes 5 cups

1	tablespoon canola oil, divided
1	pound lean boneless chuck, trimmed of fat and cut into 1-inch cubes
1	cup chopped onion
2	medium garlic cloves, minced
8	ounces whole mushrooms
1 1/2	cups water
1	cup dry red wine
2	teaspoons gluten-free Worcestershire sauce
1 1/2	teaspoons sugar
2	packets sodium-free, gluten-free beef bouillon granules
1/4	teaspoon ground allspice
2	medium carrots, scrubbed, halved lengthwise, and cut into 3-inch pieces (8 ounces total)
12	ounces russet potatoes, peeled (optional), and cut into 3/4-inch cubes
3/4	teaspoon salt

---

1. Heat 1 teaspoon of the oil in a Dutch oven over medium-high heat. Working in batches, brown half of the beef; set aside on separate plate. Repeat with 1 teaspoon of the oil and remaining beef; set aside. Add the remaining 1 teaspoon oil to the pan residue, cook the onions and garlic 3 minutes or until onions are brown on edges.

2. Stir in the mushrooms, water, wine, Worcestershire, sugar, bouillon, allspice, and return the beef to the onions in the Dutch oven. Bring to a boil over high heat, reduce heat, cover, and simmer 1 hour and 15 minutes.

3. Stir in the carrots and potatoes, cover, and cook 45 minutes or until beef is tender.

COOK'S TIP

For a thicker consistency, using a potato masher or large slotted spoon, mash some of the potatoes and carrots. This technique also adds flavor as well as thickness.

EXCHANGES/FOOD CHOICES
1 Starch, 2 Vegetable, 2 Lean Meat,
    1 Fat

BASIC NUTRITIONAL VALUES:

Calories	255	
Calories from Fat	70	
Total Fat	8.0	g
Saturated Fat	1.8	g
Trans Fat	0.2	g
Cholesterol	50	mg
Sodium	540	mg
Potassium	1025	mg
Total Carbohydrate	25	g
Dietary Fiber	3	g
Sugars	7	g
Protein	21	g
Phosphorus	250	mg

CHOP-FREE CHILI

Serves 4 • Serving Size: 1 1/2 cups (2 tablespoons sour cream and
1 tablespoon cilantro) • Makes 6 cups

---

  12 ounces extra-lean (93% lean) ground beef
   1 14.4-ounce package frozen pepper stir-fry vegetables
       OR 3 cups frozen peppers, 1 cup frozen diced onion
   2 14.5-ounce cans no-salt-added stewed tomatoes
   1 15-ounce can no-salt-added dark kidney beans, rinsed and drained
   2 teaspoons gluten-free Worcestershire sauce
   2 tablespoons chili powder
   1 tablespoon instant coffee granules
1 1/2 teaspoons ground cumin, divided
   2 tablespoons gluten-free ketchup
   1 tablespoon extra-virgin olive oil
 1/2 teaspoon salt (optional)

Toppings
 1/2 cup fat-free sour cream (read labels)
 1/4 cup chopped cilantro

---

1. Heat a Dutch oven over medium-high heat. Brown beef, stirring
   occasionally. Stir in the pepper mixture, tomatoes, beans, Worcestershire,
   chili powder, coffee granules, and 1 teaspoon of the cumin.

2. Bring to a boil over high heat, reduce heat, cover, and simmer 30 minutes.
   Stir in the remaining cumin, ketchup, oil, and salt. Serve topped with
   sour cream and cilantro.

COOK'S TIP	Coffee granules give the chili a deeper beefy flavor. And, as with most chilis, the flavors improve overnight.

EXCHANGES/FOOD CHOICES
1 Starch, 5 Vegetable, 2 Lean Meat,
1 1/2 Fat

BASIC NUTRITIONAL VALUES:

Calories	375	Trans Fat	0.3 g
Calories from Fat	100	Cholesterol	55 mg
Total Fat	11.0 g	Sodium	330 mg
Saturated Fat	3.2 g	Potassium	1300 mg
		Total Carbohydrate	46 g
		Dietary Fiber	11 g
		Sugars	21 g
		Protein	27 g
		Phosphorus	350 mg

SALADS

Practice Gluten Awareness
Be sure to always verify that your ingredients are gluten-free. Products do change over time; so don't assume that since a product was safe before, it will always be gluten-free.

AVOCADO-RICE SALAD

Serves 4 • Serving Size: 3/4 cup • Makes 3 cups

---

    1   cup frozen cooked brown rice, thawed
  1/2   cup grape tomatoes, quartered
  1/2   cup diced green bell pepper
  1/4   cup diced red onion
  1/4   cup chopped fresh cilantro
    1   medium garlic clove, minced
    2   tablespoons lime juice
    1   tablespoon cider vinegar
    1   tablespoon extra-virgin olive oil
  1/2   teaspoon salt
  1/2   medium ripe avocado, peeled, seeded, and chopped

---

1. In a medium bowl, combine all ingredients except avocado. Gently stir in avocado.
2. Let stand 5 minutes to absorb flavor slightly.

EXCHANGES/FOOD CHOICES		
1/2 Starch, 1 Vegetable, 1 Fat	Cholesterol	0 mg
	Sodium	300 mg
	Potassium	225 mg
BASIC NUTRITIONAL VALUES:	Total Carbohydrate	15 g
Calories	120	Dietary Fiber	3 g
Calories from Fat	65	Sugars	2 g
Total Fat	7.0 g	Protein	2 g
Saturated Fat	1.0 g	Phosphorus	60 mg
Trans Fat	0.0 g		

GARBANZO-LEMON PASTA SALAD

Serves 4 • Serving Size: 3/4 cup • Makes 3 cups

---

2 ounces dry quinoa or corn pasta

1/2 16-ounce can no-salt-added garbanzo beans, rinsed and drained

1/2 cup diced red bell pepper

2 teaspoons grated lemon rind

2 tablespoons lemon juice

2 tablespoons chopped fresh basil

2 tablespoons chopped parsley, preferably Italian

1 medium garlic clove, minced

1 tablespoon extra-virgin olive oil

1/4 teaspoon salt

1/8 teaspoon dried pepper flakes, optional

3/4 ounce freshly shredded or grated Parmesan cheese

---

1. Cook pasta according to package directions, omitting any salt or oil.
2. In a medium bowl, combine the remaining ingredients, except cheese.
3. Drain pasta in a colander and immediately run under cold water until completely cooled. Shake off excess water and stir into the bean mixture. Sprinkle with cheese and stir gently.

EXCHANGES/FOOD CHOICES		
1 1/2 Starch, 1 Fat		
	Cholesterol	5 mg
	Sodium	235 mg
	Potassium	255 mg
BASIC NUTRITIONAL VALUES:	Total Carbohydrate	24 g
Calories	170	Dietary Fiber	4 g
Calories from Fat	55	Sugars	3 g
Total Fat	6.0 g	Protein	7 g
Saturated Fat	1.5 g	Phosphorus	170 mg
Trans Fat	0.0 g		

QUINOA TABBOULEH SALAD

Serves 4 • Serving Size: 3/4 cup • Makes 3 cups

2	cups water
1/2	cup quinoa
1	medium tomato, seeded and diced
1/2	medium cucumber, peeled, seeded, and diced
1/3	cup diced red onion
1	cup finely chopped parsley
1/2	cup chopped fresh mint
2	medium garlic cloves, minced
2	tablespoons cider vinegar
1 1/2	tablespoons canola oil
1/2	teaspoon salt

---

1. Combine water and quinoa in a medium saucepan and bring to a boil. Reduce heat, cover, and simmer 10 minutes.

2. Meanwhile, combine the remaining ingredients in a medium bowl and set aside.

3. Drain quinoa in a fine-mesh sieve and run under cold water until completely cooled. Shake off excess water. Stir quinoa into the tomato mixture.

COOK'S TIP	Be sure to use a fine-mesh sieve because the quinoa is so small it will fall through the holes of a regular colander.

EXCHANGES/FOOD CHOICES
1 Starch, 1 Vegetable, 1 Fat

BASIC NUTRITIONAL VALUES:

Calories	160
Calories from Fat	65
Total Fat	7.0 g
Saturated Fat	0.6 g
Trans Fat	0.0 g
Cholesterol	0 mg
Sodium	310 mg
Potassium	380 mg
Total Carbohydrate	21 g
Dietary Fiber	4 g
Sugars	4 g
Protein	4 g
Phosphorus	140 mg

MUSTARD POTATO SALAD

Serves 4 • Serving Size: 3/4 cup • Makes 3 cups

---

4 cups water
12 ounces (about 2 medium) Yukon gold potatoes, diced
1/2 cup diced green pepper
1/3 cup diced onion
1/4 cup diced celery
1/3 cup gluten-free light mayonnaise
1 tablespoon cider vinegar
2 teaspoons prepared mustard
1/4 teaspoon salt
1/4 teaspoon black pepper

---

1. Bring water to boil in a medium saucepan. Add potatoes, return to a boil, reduce heat, and simmer uncovered 4–5 minutes or until potatoes are just tender.
2. Meanwhile, in a medium bowl, combine remaining ingredients and set aside.
3. Drain potatoes in a colander and run under cold water until completely cooled. Shake off excess water and stir into the green pepper mixture.
4. Serve within 1 hour for peak flavors.

COOK'S TIP To make ahead, combine all ingredients, except the cooked potatoes. Cover and refrigerate in two separate containers. Combine ingredients 30 minutes prior to serving.

EXCHANGES/FOOD CHOICES
1 1/2 Starch, 1/2 Fat

BASIC NUTRITIONAL VALUES:

Calories	145
Calories from Fat	45
Total Fat	5.0 g
Saturated Fat	0.7 g
Trans Fat	0.0 g
Cholesterol	5 mg
Sodium	350 mg
Potassium	445 mg
Total Carbohydrate	23 g
Dietary Fiber	3 g
Sugars	3 g
Protein	3 g
Phosphorus	105 mg

ROMAINE WITH CROUTONS AND CREAMY DILL DRESSING

Serves 4 • Serving Size: 2 cups salad plus 2 tablespoons salad
dressing • Makes 8 cups

---

  2 slices gluten-free sandwich bread, each slice cut into 16 cubes
     Cooking spray
  6 cups loosely packed torn romaine leaves (6 ounces)
1/2 medium cucumber, thinly sliced
1/2 cup thinly sliced red onion (2 ounces total)

Dressing
1/3 cup low-fat buttermilk
  3 tablespoons gluten-free light mayonnaise
  1 teaspoon cider vinegar
  2 medium garlic cloves, minced
  1 teaspoon dried dill weed
1/4 teaspoon black pepper
1/4 teaspoon salt

---

1. Lightly coat the bread cubes with cooking spray, place on baking sheet. Turn oven on 350°F (do not preheat oven), and bake 8 minutes or until lightly golden. Cool completely.
2. Meanwhile, in a small bowl whisk together the dressing ingredients.
3. In a large bowl combine the lettuce leaves, cucumber, and onion. Pour the dressing over all and toss gently until well coated. Add the bread cubes and toss gently.

| COOK'S TIP | Make several batches of croutons and freeze or store in an airtight container to keep on hand. |

EXCHANGES/FOOD CHOICES
1/2 Starch, 1 Vegetable, 1 Fat

BASIC NUTRITIONAL VALUES:
Calories   95
  Calories from Fat   35
Total Fat   4.0 g
  Saturated Fat   0.6 g
  Trans Fat   0.0 g

Cholesterol   5 mg
Sodium   340 mg
Potassium   305 mg
Total Carbohydrate   12 g
  Dietary Fiber   2 g
  Sugars   4 g
Protein   3 g
Phosphorus   75 mg

HERBED DIJON VINAIGRETTE

Serves 4 • Serving Size: 2 tablespoons • Makes 1/2 cup

---

   3 tablespoons extra-virgin olive oil
   3 tablespoons lemon juice or cider vinegar
   1 tablespoon Dijon mustard
   1 tablespoon water
   1 teaspoon pourable sugar substitute
   1 medium garlic clove, minced
1/2 teaspoon dried rosemary leaves
1/4 teaspoon salt
1/8 teaspoon red pepper flakes

---

1. Combine all ingredients in a small jar. Secure tightly with a lid and shake vigorously.

COOK'S TIP	May replace rosemary leaves with other herbs, such as basil, oregano, tarragon, dill, or omit completely.

EXCHANGES/FOOD CHOICES
2 Fat

BASIC NUTRITIONAL VALUES:

Calories	100
Calories from Fat	90
Total Fat	10.0 g
Saturated Fat	1.4 g
Trans Fat	0.0 g
Cholesterol	0 mg
Sodium	240 mg
Potassium	20 mg
Total Carbohydrate	2 g
Dietary Fiber	0 g
Sugars	1 g
Protein	0 g
Phosphorus	5 mg

CHICKEN-PECAN SALAD WRAPS

Serves 4 • Serving Size: 1 cup chicken mixture and 3 lettuce leaves •
Makes 4 cups chicken mixture plus 12 romaine lettuce leaves

1	medium celery stalk with leaves, thinly sliced
1/2	cup diced red bell pepper
1/2	cup diced red onion
1/4	cup gluten-free light mayonnaise
1	8-ounce can sliced water chestnuts, drained and coarsely chopped
2	ounces chopped pecans, toasted
1 1/2	tablespoons pourable sugar substitute
1	teaspoon curry powder, optional
1/4	teaspoon ground cumin
1/8–1/4	teaspoon dried pepper flakes
1/2	teaspoon salt
2	cups cooked chopped chicken breast meat
12	Romaine lettuce leaves

---

1. In a medium bowl, stir together all ingredients, except the chicken and
   lettuce. Gently stir in the chicken until well blended. Spoon equal amounts
   (about 1/3 cup) of the chicken mixture down the center of each lettuce leaf.

COOK'S TIP	May replace rosemary leaves with other herbs, such as basil, oregano, tarragon, dill, or omit completely.

EXCHANGES/FOOD CHOICES
2 Vegetable, 3 Lean Meat, 2 1/2 Fat

BASIC NUTRITIONAL VALUES:

Calories	300	Cholesterol	65 mg
Calories from Fat	155	Sodium	495 mg
Total Fat	17.0 g	Potassium	530 mg
Saturated Fat	2.1 g	Total Carbohydrate	13 g
Trans Fat	0.0 g	Dietary Fiber	5 g
		Sugars	5 g
		Protein	25 g
		Phosphorus	245 mg

NEW-FASHIONED EGG SALAD

Serves 4 • Serving Size: 1/2 cup plus 9 crackers • Makes 2 cups egg salad plus 36 crackers

---

  6 hard-boiled large eggs, peeled
  3 tablespoons gluten-free light mayonnaise
  1 teaspoon Dijon mustard
  1 teaspoon pourable sugar substitute
1/8 teaspoon salt
1/8 teaspoon black pepper
  1 medium celery stalk, finely chopped
 36 gluten-free crackers, such as rosemary and olive oil

---

1. Cut the eggs in half and discard 6 egg yolk halves. Place the remaining egg yolk halves in a medium bowl, mash with a fork, and stir in the mayonnaise, mustard, sugar substitute, salt, and black pepper.
2. Finely chop the egg whites and stir into the egg mixture with the celery. Serve with crackers.

EXCHANGES/FOOD CHOICES			Cholesterol	140 mg
1 Starch, 1 Med-Fat Meat			Sodium	435 mg
			Potassium	195 mg
BASIC NUTRITIONAL VALUES:			Total Carbohydrate	20 g
Calories	165		Dietary Fiber	2 g
Calories from Fat	55		Sugars	3 g
Total Fat	6.0 g		Protein	9 g
Saturated Fat	1.5 g		Phosphorus	155 mg
Trans Fat	0.0 g			

MAIN DISHES

Practice Gluten Awareness
Be sure to always verify that your ingredients are gluten-free. Products do
change over time; so don't assume that since a product was safe before,
it will always be gluten-free.

GARLIC-THYME CHICKEN STRIPS

Serves 4 • Serving Size: 2 chicken tenderloins and 2 tablespoons
sauce • Makes 8 chicken tenderloins and 1/2 cup sauce

- 1/2 cup 1%-fat buttermilk
- 1/4 cup egg substitute OR 2 large egg whites
- 8 chicken tenders (about 1 pound total), rinsed and patted dry
- 2/3 cup gluten-free, all-purpose baking flour, such as Bob's Red Mill
- 2 teaspoons garlic powder
- 1 teaspoon onion powder
- 1 teaspoon paprika
- 1/2 teaspoon dried thyme leaves
- 1/8 teaspoon cayenne pepper
- 1/4 teaspoon black pepper
- 1/4 teaspoon salt
- 2 tablespoons canola oil

Sauce
- 2 tablespoons gluten-free light mayonnaise
- 2 tablespoons nonfat plain Greek yogurt
- 1/4 cup apricot fruit spread
- 1 tablespoon Dijon mustard

---

1. Whisk together the buttermilk and eggs in a medium bowl, add the chicken, and toss to coat completely.
2. Place the flour, garlic powder, onion powder, paprika, thyme, cayenne, and black pepper, and 1/4 teaspoon of the salt in a shallow pan, such as a pie pan, and stir until well blended.
3. Working with two tenderloins at a time, remove from the buttermilk, coat with flour mixture, and set aside on separate plate. Continue until all tenderloins are coated. Sprinkle any remaining flour mixture evenly over all.
4. Heat the oil in a large nonstick skillet over medium-high heat until hot. Add the chicken and immediately reduce heat to medium. Cook 6 minutes on each side or until golden and no longer pink in center. Sprinkle with remaining 1/4 teaspoon salt.
5. In a small bowl, combine the sauce ingredients. Serve sauce alongside for dipping.

EXCHANGES/FOOD CHOICES
2 Carbohydrate, 4 Lean Meat, 1 Fat

BASIC NUTRITIONAL VALUES:

Calories	350
Calories from Fat	115
Total Fat	13.0 g
Saturated Fat	1.7 g
Trans Fat	0.0 g
Cholesterol	70 mg
Sodium	425 mg
Potassium	420 mg
Total Carbohydrate	30 g
Dietary Fiber	3 g
Sugars	12 g
Protein	30 g
Phosphorus	275 mg

ROASTED CHICKEN WITH DEEP ONION-GARLIC GRAVY

Serves 6 • Serving Size: 3 1/2 ounces cooked chicken and
1/4 cup gravy • Makes 21 ounces cooked chicken and 1 1/2 cups gravy

---

  2 medium onions (4 ounces each) cut in 8 wedges each
  1 garlic head (about 12–14 garlic cloves total), peeled only
  2 teaspoons paprika
  2 teaspoons dried thyme leaves
  1 teaspoon dried rosemary, crumbled
1/2 teaspoon black pepper
4- to 4 1/2-pound whole roasting chicken, cavity rinsed and patted dry
  1 tablespoon canola oil
  1 cup cold water
  2 teaspoons cornstarch
1/2 teaspoon salt

---

1. Preheat oven to 425°F.

2. Place the onions and garlic on the bottom of a 13-inch by 9-inch baking pan.

3. In a small bowl, combine the paprika, thyme, rosemary, and pepper. Coat the chicken with the oil and sprinkle the paprika mixture evenly over the chicken. Place on top of the onions and garlic. Bake 60–70 minutes or until internal temperature reaches 165°F when tested with a meat thermometer. Remove the chicken with 2 large spoons, preferably slotted, and place on cutting board. Let stand 10 minutes before slicing, discarding the skin.

4. Meanwhile, to "degrease" the pan drippings, add the cold water to the pan drippings. Stir until well blended and drain the pan residue through a fine-mesh sieve, reserving both the liquid and the strained onion mixture. Pour the liquid portion into a resealable plastic sandwich bag, seal tightly, and place in freezer for 15 minutes to allow the fat to rise to the top.

5. Hold the bag over a small saucepan. Using scissors, cut about 1/4 inch off of the corner of the bag, allowing the juices to pour into the saucepan. Stop the flow to prevent the fat from being released. Discard the bag with the fat. Stir in the cornstarch and salt until cornstarch is completely dissolved. Add the reserved onion mixture. Bring to a boil over medium-high heat. Boil 1 minute, stirring frequently. Serve with the sliced chicken.

EXCHANGES/FOOD CHOICES
4 Lean Meat

BASIC NUTRITIONAL VALUES:

Calories	195
Calories from Fat	65
Total Fat	7.0 g
Saturated Fat	2.0 g
Trans Fat	0.0 g

Cholesterol	90 mg
Sodium	280 mg
Potassium	250 mg
Total Carbohydrate	1 g
Dietary Fiber	0 g
Sugars	0 g
Protein	29 g
Phosphorus	195 mg

ITALIAN VEGGIE AND PEPPERONI PASTA

Serves 4 • Serving Size: 1 1/2 cups • Makes 6 cups

KID FRIENDLY

4	ounces uncooked gluten-free penne pasta
1	tablespoon extra-virgin olive oil, divided
1	medium green bell pepper, thinly sliced
1/2	cup diced onion
1	medium zucchini, halved lengthwise and thinly sliced
2	medium garlic cloves, minced
1	14.5-ounce can no-salt-added diced tomatoes
2	ounces turkey pepperoni, halved
1/4	cup chopped fresh basil
2 1/2	ounces reduced-fat feta, crumbled

1. Cook pasta according to package directions, omitting any salt or fat.

2. Meanwhile, heat 1 teaspoon of the oil in a large nonstick skillet over medium-high heat. Cook the peppers and onions 3 minutes or until onions are translucent. Stir in the zucchini and cook 2 minutes; add garlic and cook 15 seconds, stirring constantly. Add tomatoes and their liquid, simmer uncovered 6 minutes or until most liquid is absorbed.

3. Remove from heat. Add pepperoni, basil, and remaining 2 teaspoons oil. Spoon over drained pasta and top with feta.

COOK'S TIP	Some sausages contain gluten; here's a recipe that's safe . . . and fun!

EXCHANGES/FOOD CHOICES
1 1/2 Starch, 2 Vegetable,
1 Med-Fat Meat

BASIC NUTRITIONAL VALUES:

		Trans Fat	0.0 g
		Cholesterol	25 mg
		Sodium	570 mg
		Potassium	595 mg
Calories	240	Total Carbohydrate	33 g
Calories from Fat	70	Dietary Fiber	4 g
Total Fat	8.0 g	Sugars	5 g
Saturated Fat	2.7 g	Protein	12 g
		Phosphorus	295 mg

OVEN-FRIED CATFISH WITH CORNMEAL

Serves 4 • Serving Size: 1 fillet (3 ounces cooked fish) • Makes 4 fish fillets

---

Cooking spray
2 catfish fillets (about 8 ounces each), cut in half lengthwise, rinsed and patted dry
1/2 cup fat-free or low-fat buttermilk
1/2 cup stone ground cornmeal
1 teaspoon paprika powder
1/2 teaspoon onion powder
1/2 teaspoon garlic powder
1/4 teaspoon cayenne pepper
1/4 teaspoon salt
1 medium lemon, quartered

---

1. Preheat the oven to 425°F. Line a large baking sheet with aluminum foil. Lightly spray with cooking spray.

2. In a medium bowl, combine the fish and the buttermilk. Toss gently to coat thoroughly. Set aside.

3. Meanwhile, in a pie plate or shallow bowl, stir together the cornmeal and remaining ingredients, except salt and lemon. Set the bowl with the fish, the pie plate with the cornmeal, and the baking sheet in a row, assembly-line fashion. Working with one fish strip at a time, coat the fish with the crumbs, gently shaking off any excess. Place on the baking sheet. Lightly coat the top of the fish with cooking spray.

4. Bake for 12 minutes, or until the fish is golden brown and flakes easily when tested with a fork. Remove from the oven and sprinkle evenly with the salt. Serve with lemon wedges.

EXCHANGES/FOOD CHOICES		
1 Starch, 3 Lean Meat	Cholesterol	65 mg
	Sodium	290 mg
	Potassium	450 mg
BASIC NUTRITIONAL VALUES:	Total Carbohydrate	13 g
Calories 210	Dietary Fiber	1 g
Calories from Fat 70	Sugars	2 g
Total Fat 8.0 g	Protein	21 g
Saturated Fat 1.7 g	Phosphorus	285 mg
Trans Fat 0.1 g		

SHRIMP AND RICE NOODLES, PAD-THAI STYLE

Serves 4 • Serving Size: 1 1/2 cups • Makes 6 cups

---

    4 ounces uncooked flat rice noodles
    5 ounces uncooked peeled shrimp
    1 cup matchstick carrots
   12 ounces asparagus spears, cut into 1-inch pieces
    1 cup chopped green onion (white and green parts total)
    1 medium lime, quartered

Sauce
   1/2 cup plus 2 tablespoons chopped fresh cilantro, divided
     1 medium jalapeño, halved lengthwise (and seeded, optional)
     1 tablespoon minced peeled gingerroot
   1/3 cup gluten-free low-sodium, 33%-less-sugar peanut butter, such as Jif
     2 tablespoons pourable sugar substitute
     3 tablespoons water
 1 1/2 tablespoons lime juice
 1 1/2 tablespoons plain rice vinegar or white vinegar
 1 1/2 tablespoons gluten-free, reduced-sodium soy sauce

---

1. Cook noodles according to package directions, about 5 minutes.
   Add shrimp and cook for 1 minute, then add the carrots and asparagus,
   and cook for 2 minutes longer or until vegetables are just tender-crisp.

2. Meanwhile, in a blender, combine all the sauce ingredients, except
   2 tablespoons of the cilantro, purée until smooth, and set aside.

3. Drain the noodle mixture in colander, shaking off excess liquid. Place in
   a shallow pasta bowl. Pour the sauce over all, top with the green onions,
   and toss until well blended. Sprinkle with the remaining 2 tablespoons
   cilantro and garnish with a lime wedge.

EXCHANGES/FOOD CHOICES

1 1/2 Starch, 2 Vegetable, 1 Lean
   Meat, 2 Fat

BASIC NUTRITIONAL VALUES:

Calories	305
Calories from Fat	100
Total Fat	11.0 g
Saturated Fat	1.8 g
Trans Fat	0.0 g
Cholesterol	45 mg
Sodium	600 mg
Potassium	605 mg
Total Carbohydrate	40 g
Dietary Fiber	5 g
Sugars	7 g
Protein	14 g
Phosphorus	260 mg

COD ON ROASTED PEPPER AND WHITE BEANS

Serves 4 • Serving Size: 3 ounces cooked fish and 1/2 cup bean
mixture • Makes 4 fillets and 2 cups bean mixture

Fish
- 1/2 teaspoon paprika
- 1/4 teaspoon salt
- 1/4 teaspoon black pepper
- 4 5-ounce fish fillets, such as cod, rinsed and patted dry
- 1 teaspoon extra-virgin olive oil

Beans
- 1/4 cup water
- 1 15-ounce can no-salt-added navy beans or Great Northern, rinsed and drained
- 16 pitted kalamata olives, coarsely chopped
- 1/2 cup diced roasted red peppers
- 2 medium garlic cloves, minced
- 2 teaspoons extra-virgin olive oil
- 1/2 teaspoon chopped fresh rosemary or to taste
- 1/8 teaspoon salt

---

1. In a small bowl, combine the paprika, 1/4 teaspoon of the salt, and black pepper. Sprinkle both sides of the fillets with the paprika mixture. Heat 1 teaspoon of the oil in a large nonstick skillet over medium heat. Cook the fillets 4 minutes, turn, and cook 3 minutes or until opaque in center.

2. Meanwhile, bring the water to a boil over medium-high heat in a medium saucepan. Add the remaining bean ingredients. Cook 1–2 minutes to heat through. Remove from heat, cover, and let stand while fish is cooking.

3. To serve, place equal amounts of the bean mixture in each of 4 shallow soup bowls or rimmed dinner plates, top with the fillets.

EXCHANGES/FOOD CHOICES
1 Starch, 4 Lean Meat

BASIC NUTRITIONAL VALUES:

Calories	285
Calories from Fat	80
Total Fat	9.0 g
Saturated Fat	1.1 g
Trans Fat	0.0 g
Cholesterol	60 mg
Sodium	505 mg
Potassium	490 mg
Total Carbohydrate	21 g
Dietary Fiber	7 g
Sugars	2 g
Protein	32 g
Phosphorus	260 mg

BLACK BEAN QUINOA PILAF WITH FETA

Serves 4 • Serving Size: 1 1/4 cups • Makes 5 cups

1/4 cup plus 2 tablespoons instant brown rice
1/4 cup dry quinoa
1 cup plus 2 tablespoons water
1 tablespoon canola oil, divided
8 ounces whole mushrooms, quartered
1 cup diced onion
1 cup diced green bell pepper
1/2 15-ounce can no-salt-added black beans, rinsed and drained
2 medium garlic cloves, minced
1 ounce pine nuts, toasted
1/4 cup chopped fresh parsley
1/2 teaspoon salt
3 ounces reduced-fat feta, crumbled

---

1. In a medium saucepan, combine the rice, quinoa, and water. Bring to a boil, reduce heat, cover tightly, and simmer 10 minutes or until water is absorbed.

2. Meanwhile, heat 1 teaspoon of the oil in a large nonstick skillet over medium-high heat. Cook the mushrooms 4 minutes or until beginning to lightly brown, stirring occasionally. Add the onions and peppers to the mushrooms and cook 4 minutes or until onions are beginning to brown on the edges, stirring occasionally.

3. Remove from the heat, stir in the remaining ingredients, except the feta. Sprinkle with the feta.

EXCHANGES/FOOD CHOICES
1 1/2 Starch, 2 Vegetable,
1 Med-Fat Meat, 1 Fat

BASIC NUTRITIONAL VALUES:

Calories	295	
Calories from Fat	115	
Total Fat	13.0	g
Saturated Fat	2.7	g
Trans Fat	0.0	g
Cholesterol	5	mg
Sodium	600	mg
Potassium	620	mg
Total Carbohydrate	35	g
Dietary Fiber	6	g
Sugars	5	g
Protein	13	g
Phosphorus	325	mg

MAKE-AHEAD MARINARA SAUCE

Serves 16 • Serving Size: 1/2 cup • Makes 8 cups

---

2 tablespoons extra-virgin olive oil, divided
2 cups diced yellow onion
8 garlic cloves, minced
4 14.5-ounce cans no-salt-added diced tomatoes
2 6-ounce cans gluten-free, no-salt-added tomato paste (check labels)
2 teaspoons sugar
2 teaspoons dried oregano leaves
1 large bay leaf
1/4 teaspoon dried red pepper flakes
1/2 cup chopped fresh basil
1 teaspoon salt

---

1. Heat 1 teaspoon of the oil in a Dutch oven over medium heat. Cook the onions 6 minutes, or until translucent. Add the garlic and cook 30 seconds, stirring constantly. Stir in the tomatoes, tomato paste, sugar, oregano, bay leaf, and pepper flakes. Bring to a boil, reduce heat, cover, and simmer 1 hour. Remove and discard bay leaf after cooking.

2. Remove Dutch oven from heat, stir in the basil, salt, and remaining oil. Cover and let stand at least 10 minutes.

| COOK'S TIP | Flavor improves overnight. Not only is this is a great make-ahead recipe, it is also a great freezer recipe to keep on hand. It's safer (and tastier) to make marinara from scratch rather than purchase the prepared variety because many store-bought sauces contain gluten. |

EXCHANGES/FOOD CHOICES		Cholesterol	0 mg
2 Vegetable, 1/2 Fat		Sodium	210 mg
		Potassium	450 mg
BASIC NUTRITIONAL VALUES:		Total Carbohydrate	11 g
Calories	65	Dietary Fiber	2 g
Calories from Fat	20	Sugars	6 g
Total Fat	2.0 g	Protein	2 g
Saturated Fat	0.3 g	Phosphorus	45 mg
Trans Fat	0.0 g		

SIRLOIN STEAK WITH DEEP BALSAMIC REDUCTION

Serves 4 • Serving Size: 3 ounces cooked beef and 1 1/2 teaspoons sauce • Makes 12 ounces beef and 2 tablespoons sauce

1	pound trimmed boneless sirloin steak (about 3/4 inch thick)
1/4	cup balsamic vinegar
1/4	cup water
1	tablespoon pourable sugar substitute
2	teaspoons coffee granules
1	teaspoon dried oregano leaves
1/2	teaspoon garlic powder
1/4	teaspoon onion powder
1/2	teaspoon black pepper
1/4	teaspoon red pepper flakes
	Cooking spray
1/4	teaspoon salt

1. Place the steak in a gallon-size resealable plastic bag. In a small bowl, combine the vinegar, water, sugar substitute, coffee granules, oregano, garlic powder, onion powder, black pepper, and pepper flakes. Pour half of the mixture over the steak and seal. Toss back and forth and refrigerate 8 hours or up to 48 hours, turning occasionally. Cover and refrigerate remaining marinade.

2. Heat a grill pan coated with cooking spray over medium-high heat. Remove the beef from the bag, discard the marinade in the bag, and cook 4 minutes on each side or to desired doneness. Place on cutting board and let stand 3 minutes before thinly slicing.

3. Meanwhile, place the reserved marinade and the salt in a small saucepan. Bring to a boil over high heat and boil 1 1/2–2 minutes or until reduced to 2 tablespoons. Drizzle over sliced beef.

COOK'S TIP	The sauce is very concentrated. Just a small amount is all that is needed.

EXCHANGES/FOOD CHOICES
3 Lean Meat

BASIC NUTRITIONAL VALUES:

Calories	150
Calories from Fat	40
Total Fat	4.5 g
Saturated Fat	1.6 g
Trans Fat	0.1 g

Cholesterol	40 mg
Sodium	195 mg
Potassium	325 mg
Total Carbohydrate	3 g
Dietary Fiber	0 g
Sugars	2 g
Protein	23 g
Phosphorus	185 mg

WORRY-FREE AND DOWN-HOME MEATLOAF

Serves 4 • Serving Size: 1/4 recipe • Makes 1 meatloaf

KID FRIENDLY

1	pound extra-lean (93% lean) ground beef
2/3	cup gluten-free rolled oats
1/2	cup diced green bell pepper
1/2	cup diced onion
3	egg whites
1	8-ounce can gluten-free, no-salt-added tomato sauce, divided
1/2	teaspoon dried thyme leaves
1/2	teaspoon salt
1/2	teaspoon black pepper
	Cooking spray
2	teaspoons pourable sugar substitute
1	tablespoon balsamic vinegar

1. Preheat oven to 350°F.

2. Combine the beef, oats, bell pepper, onion, egg whites, 1/2 cup of the tomato sauce, thyme, 1/4 teaspoon of the salt, and black pepper in a medium bowl. Coat a foil-lined baking sheet with cooking spray, place the beef mixture on the baking sheet, and shape into an oval (about 5 inches by 8 inches and about 1 1/2–2 inches thick).

3. Combine the remaining tomato sauce with the remaining ingredients in a small bowl and spoon all but 2 tablespoons of the sauce evenly over the top and down the sides of the meatloaf. Bake 50 minutes or until no longer pink in center and internal temperature reaches 160°F. Spoon reserved 2 tablespoons sauce evenly over the meatloaf and let stand 10 minutes before slicing.

COOK'S TIP	Be careful when purchasing oats. Check the label and make sure to buy uncontaminated, gluten-free oats. Many brands process the oats in a facility where they also process wheat, soy, and egg products.

EXCHANGES/FOOD CHOICES
1 Starch, 1 Vegetable, 3 Lean Meat,
 1 Fat

BASIC NUTRITIONAL VALUES:

Calories	275
Calories from Fat	80
Total Fat	9.0 g
Saturated Fat	3.4 g
Trans Fat	0.4 g
Cholesterol	70 mg
Sodium	275 mg
Potassium	690 mg
Total Carbohydrate	19 g
Dietary Fiber	4 g
Sugars	5 g
Protein	28 g
Phosphorus	300 mg

BEEF AND EGGPLANT WITH FRESH MINT

Serves 4 • Serving Size: 2 eggplant slices, 1/2 cup beef mixture, 2 tablespoons mint, and 2 tablespoons cheese • Makes 8 eggplant slices, 2 cups beef mixture, 1/2 cup mint, and 1/2 cup cheese mixture

---

1	teaspoon canola oil
8	ounces extra-lean ground beef
1	cup diced onion
1	cup diced red bell pepper
1	pound eggplant, cut in 8 slices
1	8-ounce can no-salt tomato sauce
1/4	cup water
1	teaspoon ground cinnamon
1/2	teaspoon ground cumin
1/4	teaspoon dried pepper flakes, optional
1/2	teaspoon salt
2	ounces slivered almonds, toasted
1 1/2	teaspoons packed Splenda Brown Sugar Blend
1/3	cup nonfat plain Greek yogurt
1	ounce goat cheese
1/2	cup chopped fresh mint

---

1. Preheat broiler.
2. Heat the oil in a large nonstick skillet over medium-high heat. Brown the beef, stirring frequently. Add the onion and peppers. Cook 5–6 minutes or until onions are translucent. Stir in the tomato sauce, water, cinnamon, cumin, pepper flakes, and salt. Cover and cook 15 minutes or until onions are tender. Stir almonds and Splenda Brown Sugar Blend into beef mixture.
3. Meanwhile, coat a nonstick baking sheet with cooking spray, arrange eggplant slices on baking sheet, and lightly spray both sides of eggplant slices with cooking spray. Broil no closer than 5–6 inches away from heat source for 5 minutes, then turn and broil 4–5 minutes or until lightly brown and tender.
4. Place the goat cheese in a small bowl and microwave on high for 15 seconds to soften slightly; whisk in the yogurt until well blended.
5. To serve, top eggplant slices with equal amounts of the beef mixture, sprinkle with mint, and top with equal amounts of the yogurt mixture.

EXCHANGES/FOOD CHOICES
4 Vegetable, 2 Lean Meat, 2 1/2 Fat

BASIC NUTRITIONAL VALUES:

Calories	305	
Calories from Fat	135	
Total Fat	15.0	g
Saturated Fat	3.5	g
Trans Fat	0.2	g
Cholesterol	40	mg
Sodium	385	mg
Potassium	785	mg
Total Carbohydrate	26	g
Dietary Fiber	8	g
Sugars	11	g
Protein	20	g
Phosphorus	265	mg

TEX-MEX STUFFED PEPPERS

Serves 4 • Serving Size: 1 stuffed pepper • Makes 4 stuffed peppers

---

1	tablespoon canola oil
8	ounces extra-lean (93% lean) ground beef
1/2	cup diced onion
1	14.5-ounce can no-salt-added stewed tomatoes, drained, reserving liquid
1/2	cup frozen corn kernels, thawed
1/2	15-ounce can no-salt-added kidney or pinto beans, rinsed and drained
2	ounces gluten-free tortilla chips, coarsely crumbled
1	tablespoon chili powder
1	teaspoon ground cumin
1/2	teaspoon salt
4	medium green bell peppers
1	ounce shredded reduced-fat sharp cheddar cheese
1/2	cup water

---

1. Preheat oven to 350°F.
2. Heat oil in a large nonstick skillet over medium-high heat. Cook beef until browned. Add onions to the beef and cook 3 minutes or until translucent, stirring frequently. Add the tomatoes, 1/2 cup of the reserved liquid, corn, beans, tortilla chips, chili powder, cumin, and salt. Remove skillet from heat.
3. Cut the tops off of the peppers and discard seeds. Spoon equal amounts of the tomato mixture into each pepper, pressing down to pack tightly. Place stuffed peppers in a 13-inch by 9-inch baking pan; pour the remaining reserved liquid and water in bottom of pan. Cover and bake 1 hour or until peppers are tender. Top with cheese.

EXCHANGES/FOOD CHOICES			
1 1/2 Starch, 2 Vegetable, 2 Lean Meat, 2 1/2 Fat		Trans Fat	0.2 g
		Cholesterol	40 mg
		Sodium	505 mg
		Potassium	945 mg
BASIC NUTRITIONAL VALUES:		Total Carbohydrate	37 g
Calories	330	Dietary Fiber	9 g
Calories from Fat	115	Sugars	12 g
Total Fat	13.0 g	Protein	20 g
Saturated Fat	3.3 g	Phosphorus	290 mg

VERSATILE FREEZABLE MEATBALLS

Serves 4 • Serving Size: 8 meatballs (for main course) • Makes 32 meatballs

KID FRIENDLY

1 pound extra-lean (93% lean) ground beef
1/2 cup gluten-free rolled oats
1/3 cup finely chopped onion
2 medium jalapeños, finely chopped (with seeds, optional)
1/4 cup finely chopped parsley
2 medium garlic cloves, minced
2 egg whites
1/4 teaspoon salt
1 teaspoon canola oil

1. In a medium bowl, combine all the ingredients, except the oil. Shape into 32 balls (about 1 tablespoon each).
2. Heat the oil in a large nonstick skillet over medium-high heat. Cook the meatballs 10 minutes or until no longer pink in center, gently turning occasionally.
3. Serve warm or cool completely and freeze in an airtight container up to 1 month.

COOK'S TIP	This is great to add to gluten-free spaghetti sauce with gluten-free pasta or gluten-free Italian bread or to serve as an appetizer with your favorite gluten-free gravy or sauce.

EXCHANGES/FOOD CHOICES
1/2 Starch, 1 Vegetable, 3 Lean Meat, 1 Fat

BASIC NUTRITIONAL VALUES:

Calories	250	Trans Fat	0.4 g
Calories from Fat	90	Cholesterol	70 mg
Total Fat	10.0 g	Sodium	245 mg
Saturated Fat	3.4 g	Potassium	530 mg
		Total Carbohydrate	12 g
		Dietary Fiber	2 g
		Sugars	2 g
		Protein	26 g
		Phosphorus	270 mg

PORK CHOPS WITH TOMATO-TOPPED AU JUS

Serves 4 • Serving Size: 3 ounces pork and 2 tablespoons sauce •
Makes 4 pork chops and 1/2 cup sauce

1	teaspoon dried thyme leaves
1/2	teaspoon garlic powder
1/2	teaspoon black pepper
4	boneless pork chops, trimmed of fat (1 pound total)
1	tablespoon extra-virgin olive oil, divided
2/3	cup water
1	teaspoon instant coffee granules
1	teaspoon gluten-free Worcestershire sauce
1/2	teaspoon salt
1	medium tomato, seeded and diced (about 4 ounces)

---

1. In a small bowl, combine the thyme, garlic powder, and black pepper.
   Sprinkle both sides of the pork chops with the thyme mixture. Heat
   1 teaspoon of the oil in a medium nonstick skillet over medium-high heat
   until hot. Cook the pork 5 minutes, turn, and cook 4–5 minutes or until
   slightly pink in center.

2. Meanwhile, combine the water, coffee granules, Worcestershire, and salt
   in a small bowl and set aside.

3. Place the pork chops on a plate. Cover to keep warm. Add the Worcestershire mixture to the skillet and bring to a boil over medium-high heat. Boil
   4 minutes or until reduced to 1/4 cup. Stir in the tomatoes and remaining
   2 teaspoons of the oil. Cook 30 seconds. Spoon evenly over the pork chops.

COOK'S TIP	Don't cook the tomatoes longer than 30 seconds. You want to retain the shape, texture, and bright color of the toma-toes! This recipe yields enough sauce to serve with 2 cups of mashed potatoes or rice.

EXCHANGES/FOOD CHOICES
3 Lean Meat, 1 Fat

BASIC NUTRITIONAL VALUES:

Calories	195
Calories from Fat	100
Total Fat	11.0 g
Saturated Fat	3.0 g
Trans Fat	0.0 g
Cholesterol	60 mg
Sodium	355 mg
Potassium	385 mg
Total Carbohydrate	2 g
Dietary Fiber	0 g
Sugars	1 g
Protein	21 g
Phosphorus	185 mg

SLOW-SMOTHERED PORK CHOPS

Serves 4 • Serving Size: 3 ounces pork and 1/4 cup gravy • Makes 4 pork chops and 1 cup sauce

---

1/4	teaspoon paprika
1/4	teaspoon dried thyme leaves
1/2	teaspoon black pepper
4	4-ounce boneless pork chops
2 1/2	tablespoons canola oil, divided
2	tablespoons gluten-free flour
1 1/2	cups gluten-free, reduced-sodium chicken broth
1/2	teaspoon salt

---

1. Combine the paprika, thyme, and black pepper in a small bowl. Sprinkle evenly over both sides of the pork chops. Heat 1 1/2 teaspoons of the oil in a medium nonstick skillet over medium-high heat. Cook the pork chops 3 minutes on each side or until browned. Set aside on separate plate.

2. Whisk together the flour and remaining oil in the skillet and cook 1 minute, stirring constantly. Gradually whisk in the broth. Return the pork chops and any accumulated juices to the skillet. Bring to a boil over medium heat, cover, reduce heat, and simmer 30 minutes or until pork is tender. Remove pork chops and place on serving plate. Stir in the salt using a flat spatula to scrape up any browned bits. Spoon sauce over all.

COOK'S TIP	There is enough sauce to serve with 2 cups of mashed potatoes or rice alongside.

EXCHANGES/FOOD CHOICES
3 Lean Meat, 2 Fat

BASIC NUTRITIONAL VALUES:

Calories	245
Calories from Fat	155
Total Fat	17.0 g
Saturated Fat	3.5 g
Trans Fat	0.0 g

Cholesterol	45 mg
Sodium	515 mg
Potassium	385 mg
Total Carbohydrate	3 g
Dietary Fiber	1 g
Sugars	0 g
Protein	20 g
Phosphorus	180 mg

SO FAST SALSA VERDE PORK AND RICE CASSEROLE

Serves 4 • Serving Size: 1 cup and 2 tablespoons sour cream • Makes 4 cups

---

1	teaspoon canola oil
1	pound boneless pork chops, thinly sliced
1	teaspoon ground cumin
1 1/2	cups water
3/4	cup instant brown rice
1/2	cup tomatillo sauce (salsa verde)
2	ounces shredded reduced-fat Mexican four-cheese or reduced-fat sharp cheddar cheese (optional)
1/4	cup chopped cilantro
1/2	cup grape tomatoes, quartered
1/2	cup fat-free sour cream (read labels)
1	medium lime, quartered

---

1. Heat the oil in large nonstick skillet over medium-high heat. Add the pork to the skillet, sprinkle with cumin, and cook 2–3 minutes or until slightly pink in center. Set aside on separate plate.

2. To pan residue add rice and water. Bring to boil over medium-high heat, reduce, cover, and simmer 10 minutes. Remove from heat, stir in the pork, top with the tomatillo sauce, and sprinkle cheese and tomatoes over all. Cover and let stand 5 minutes to absorb flavors. Sprinkle with the cilantro and serve with sour cream and lime wedges.

EXCHANGES/FOOD CHOICES		
1 Starch, 1/2 Carbohydrate, 3 Lean Meat, 1 Fat		
	Trans Fat	0.0 g
	Cholesterol	60 mg
	Sodium	275 mg
	Potassium	530 mg
BASIC NUTRITIONAL VALUES:	Total Carbohydrate	28 g
Calories	300	Dietary Fiber	2 g
Calories from Fat	80	Sugars	3 g
Total Fat	9.0 g	Protein	25 g
Saturated Fat	2.8 g	Phosphorus	300 mg

SIDES

Practice Gluten Awareness
Be sure to always verify that your ingredients are gluten-free. Products do change over time; so don't assume that since a product was safe before, it will always be gluten-free.

LEMON-DILL RICE

Serves 4 • Serving Size: 1/2 cup • Makes 2 cups

---

1 1/4	cups water
3/4	cup instant brown rice
1	tablespoon extra-virgin olive oil
2	teaspoons grated lemon rind
1 1/2	teaspoons chopped fresh dill OR 1/2 teaspoon dried dill weed
1/2	teaspoon salt

---

1. In a medium saucepan, bring water to boil over high heat. Add the rice and cook according to package directions. Remove from heat, stir in remaining ingredients.

EXCHANGES/FOOD CHOICES
1 Starch, 1 Fat

BASIC NUTRITIONAL VALUES:

Calories	120	Cholesterol	0 mg
Calories from Fat	35	Sodium	300 mg
Total Fat	4.0 g	Potassium	40 mg
Saturated Fat	0.5 g	Total Carbohydrate	19 g
Trans Fat	0.0 g	Dietary Fiber	1 g
		Sugars	0 g
		Protein	2 g
		Phosphorus	75 mg

PARMESAN SCALLOPED RED POTATOES

Serves 4 • Serving Size: 3/4 cup • Makes 3 cups

---

    1 slice gluten-free bread, such as Udi's whole-grain bread, torn into
       several pieces
    1 ounce freshly grated Parmesan cheese
   12 ounces red potatoes, thinly sliced*
  3/4 cup thinly sliced onions
  2/3 cup fat-free evaporated milk
  1/8 teaspoon ground nutmeg
  1/4 teaspoon salt
  1/4 teaspoon black pepper
    1 tablespoon trans-fat-free margarine

---

1. Preheat the oven to 325°F.
2. Place the torn bread in a food processor or blender and process until a crumb texture is achieved. Place in a small bowl with the cheese, toss until well blended, and set aside.
3. Layer half of the potatoes in the bottom of a 9-inch deep-dish pie pan. Place the onions evenly over the potatoes and arrange the remaining potatoes over all.
4. In a small saucepan, combine the milk, nutmeg, salt, and pepper. Bring to a boil over medium-high heat and pour evenly over all. Place the margarine in the saucepan and stir until melted. Drizzle evenly over all. Cover and bake 30 minutes.
5. Remove the cover and sprinkle the reserved bread crumb mixture evenly over all. Bake, uncovered, 20 minutes or until potatoes are tender. Let stand 5 minutes to thicken slightly and allow flavors to blend.

*This may be done by hand or in a food processor.

EXCHANGES/FOOD CHOICES
1 Starch, 1/2 Fat-Free Milk, 1/2 Fat

BASIC NUTRITIONAL VALUES:

Calories	160	Cholesterol	5 mg
Calories from Fat	35	Sodium	380 mg
		Potassium	605 mg
Total Fat	4.0 g	Total Carbohydrate	23 g
Saturated Fat	1.7 g	Dietary Fiber	2 g
Trans Fat	0.0 g	Sugars	7 g
		Protein	8 g
		Phosphorus	205 mg

SWEET POTATO CASSEROLE WITH GINGER STREUSEL TOPPING

Serves 10 • Serving Size: 1/2 cup • Makes about 5 1/3 cups

Base
- 2 quarts water
- 3 sweet potatoes (2 pounds), peeled and cut into 1/2-inch cubes
- 1/4 cup packed Splenda Brown Sugar Blend
- 1/4 cup trans-fat-free margarine
- 1/4 cup fat-free half-and-half
- 1/4 cup egg substitute
- 1/2 teaspoon vanilla, butter, and nut flavoring OR 1 teaspoon vanilla
- 1/2 teaspoon salt

Topping
- 8 gluten-free gingersnap cookies (1 2/3 ounces total; 6 grams each), crushed
- 1 ounce chopped pecans, preferably toasted
- 2 tablespoons packed Splenda Brown Sugar Blend
- 1 tablespoon gluten-free all-purpose flour
- 1 1/2 tablespoons canola oil

---

1. Preheat oven to 350°F.

2. Bring water to a boil in a Dutch oven over high heat. Add potatoes, return to a boil, reduce heat, cover, and simmer 10–12 minutes or until very tender.

3. Remove from the heat, drain potatoes well, and return to the Dutch oven with the remaining base ingredients. Using an electric mixer or potato masher, beat until smooth. Spoon into an 11-inch by 7-inch baking dish.

4. In a medium bowl, combine all of the topping ingredients, except the oil, and stir until well blended. Drizzle the oil over all and toss gently with a fork until crumbly. Sprinkle streusel over sweet potatoes and bake, uncovered, for 25 minutes or until streusel is lightly browned. Let stand 5 minutes to allow flavors to blend.

EXCHANGES/FOOD CHOICES
1 Starch, 1 Carbohydrate, 1 Fat

BASIC NUTRITIONAL VALUES:

Calories	185
Calories from Fat	65
Total Fat	7.0 g
Saturated Fat	1.1 g
Trans Fat	0.0 g

Cholesterol	0 mg
Sodium	205 mg
Potassium	270 mg
Total Carbohydrate	27 g
Dietary Fiber	3 g
Sugars	11 g
Protein	3 g
Phosphorus	55 mg

CREAMY POBLANO CORN

Serves 4 • Serving Size: 1/2 cup • Makes 2 cups

1	teaspoon canola oil
1	cup diced onion
1	medium poblano chile pepper, seeded and diced
2	cups frozen corn kernels
1 1/2	ounces soft tub light cream cheese (3 tablespoons)
3	tablespoons fat-free milk
2	tablespoons chopped cilantro
1/4	teaspoon black pepper
1/4	teaspoon salt
1/4	cup diced roasted red peppers

---

1. Heat the oil in a medium saucepan over medium heat. Cook the onion and chile for 5 minutes or until peppers are tender, stirring frequently.

2. Stir in the corn, cream cheese, and milk. Bring just to a boil over medium heat. Reduce the heat and simmer, covered, for 10 minutes or until mixture has thickened slightly and onions are very soft. Remove from the heat, let stand 5 minutes, uncovered, to absorb flavors.

3. Stir in the remaining ingredients. Sprinkle with diced roasted red peppers.

EXCHANGES/FOOD CHOICES
1 Starch, 1 Vegetable, 1/2 Fat

BASIC NUTRITIONAL VALUES:

Calories	120	Cholesterol	5 mg
Calories from Fat	35	Sodium	235 mg
Total Fat	4.0 g	Potassium	335 mg
Saturated Fat	1.4 g	Total Carbohydrate	21 g
Trans Fat	0.0 g	Dietary Fiber	3 g
		Sugars	6 g
		Protein	4 g
		Phosphorus	105 mg

JALAPEÑO-CHEESE GRITS

Serves 4 • Serving Size: 1/2 cup • Makes 2 cups

---

2 cups water
1/2 cup gluten-free quick-cooking grits, such as Bob's Red Mill
1/2 teaspoon garlic powder
3/8 teaspoon salt

Topping
1 tablespoon finely chopped fresh parsley
1 1/2 ounces shredded reduced-fat sharp cheddar cheese
1 medium jalapeño, seeded and finely chopped
1/4 cup diced tomatoes OR 1/4 cup grape tomatoes, diced

---

1. Combine water, grits, and garlic powder in a medium saucepan; bring to a boil over high heat. Reduce heat, cover, and simmer 5 minutes or until thickened. Remove from heat and stir in salt. Top with parsley, cheddar cheese, tomatoes, and jalapeño.

EXCHANGES/FOOD CHOICES
1 Starch, 1/2 Fat

BASIC NUTRITIONAL VALUES:

Calories	100
Calories from Fat	20
Total Fat	2.5 g
Saturated Fat	1.3 g
Trans Fat	0.0 g
Cholesterol	5 mg
Sodium	315 mg
Potassium	110 mg
Total Carbohydrate	16 g
Dietary Fiber	1 g
Sugars	1 g
Protein	5 g
Phosphorus	90 mg

CRUNCHY CRUMB SUMMER SQUASH CASSEROLE

Serves 6 • Serving Size: 1/2 cup • Makes 3 cups

---

    1   teaspoon canola oil
    1   cup diced onion
    1   pound yellow squash, sliced
    3   tablespoons gluten-free light mayonnaise
    3   tablespoons fat-free sour cream (read labels)
  1/4   teaspoon plus 1/8 teaspoon salt, divided
  1/8   teaspoon black pepper
  3/4   cup gluten-free corn flakes, coarsely crumbled
    2   tablespoons trans-fat-free margarine, melted

---

1. Heat the oil in a large nonstick skillet over medium heat. Cook onions 3 minutes, add squash to the onions, and cook 10 minutes or until squash is tender, stirring occasionally.

2. Remove skillet from heat, stir in the mayonnaise, sour cream, 1/4 teaspoon of the salt, and pepper. Place in an 11-inch by 7-inch casserole dish. Sprinkle evenly with the corn flakes, drizzle with the margarine, and sprinkle with remaining salt. Bake 20 minutes or until bubbly around edges. Let stand 5 minutes to absorb liquid and thicken slightly.

EXCHANGES/FOOD CHOICES
1 Vegetable, 1 Fat

BASIC NUTRITIONAL VALUES:

Calories	85	Cholesterol	5 mg
Calories from Fat	45	Sodium	270 mg
Total Fat	5.0 g	Potassium	245 mg
Saturated Fat	1.4 g	Total Carbohydrate	9 g
Trans Fat	0.0 g	Dietary Fiber	1 g
		Sugars	4 g
		Protein	2 g
		Phosphorus	45 mg

TWO-CHEESE CHEESE SAUCE

Serves 8 • Serving Size: 1 tablespoon • Makes 1/2 cup

1	tablespoon gluten-free, all-purpose baking flour
1/8	teaspoon cayenne
1	cup fat-free milk, divided
1 1/2	ounces shredded reduced-fat sharp cheddar cheese
1/2	ounce blue cheese, crumbled
1/2	teaspoon Dijon mustard
1/4	teaspoon salt

---

1. In a small saucepan, whisk together flour and cayenne with 1/4 cup of the milk. Whisk in remaining milk until smooth. Place over medium heat and cook until slightly thickened, about 3–4 minutes, stirring constantly using a flat spatula.
2. Remove from heat, stir in remaining ingredients until smooth.

COOK'S TIP This is a great sauce to serve over steamed veggies, such as broccoli, green beans, asparagus, or cauliflower.

EXCHANGES/FOOD CHOICES
1/2 Fat

BASIC NUTRITIONAL VALUES:

Calories	35
Calories from Fat	15
Total Fat	1.5 g
Saturated Fat	1.0 g
Trans Fat	0.0 g

Cholesterol	5 mg
Sodium	160 mg
Potassium	60 mg
Total Carbohydrate	2 g
Dietary Fiber	0 g
Sugars	2 g
Protein	3 g
Phosphorus	70 mg

CORN'D MUFFINS WITH BUTTERY HONEY SPREAD

Serves 12 • Serving Size: 1 muffin and 2 teaspoons spread •
Makes 12 muffins and 1/2 cup spread

Muffins

    Cooking spray
  1 cup gluten-free, all-purpose baking flour
  1 cup stone-ground yellow cornmeal
  2 tablespoons pourable sugar substitute
  2 teaspoons baking powder
1/2 teaspoon baking soda
1/2 teaspoon xanthan gum
1/4 teaspoon salt
  1 cup 1% fat buttermilk
1/4 cup egg substitute
1/4 cup canola oil
3/4 cup frozen corn kernels, thawed

Spread
1/4 cup plus 2 tablespoons gluten-free, trans-fat-free margarine
  2 tablespoons honey

1. Preheat oven to 425°F. Coat a 12-cup nonstick muffin tin with cooking spray.

2. Combine the flour, cornmeal, sugar substitute, baking powder, baking soda, xanthan gum, and salt in a medium bowl, stir until well blended.

3. Combine the remaining muffin ingredients, except the corn, in a separate medium bowl and stir until well blended. Stir in the corn.

4. Pour the buttermilk mixture into the cornmeal mixture and stir until just blended. Spoon the batter into the muffin tins. Bake 12 minutes or until wooden pick inserted comes out clean. Let stand 10 minutes before removing.

5. Meanwhile, combine the spread ingredients in a small bowl. Stir until well blended and fluffy. Serve with muffins.

EXCHANGES/FOOD CHOICES
1 1/2 Carbohydrate, 1 1/2 Fat

BASIC NUTRITIONAL VALUES:

Calories	175
Calories from Fat	70
Total Fat	8.0 g
Saturated Fat	1.2 g
Trans Fat	0.0 g
Cholesterol	0 mg
Sodium	235 mg
Potassium	125 mg
Total Carbohydrate	23 g
Dietary Fiber	2 g
Sugars	5 g
Protein	3 g
Phosphorus	135 mg

DESSERTS

Practice Gluten Awareness

Be sure to always verify that your ingredients are gluten-free. Products do change over time; so don't assume that since a product was safe before, it will always be gluten-free.

APPLE-CINNAMON PIE

Serves 8 • Serving Size: 1 slice • Makes one 9-inch pie

Filling
- 4 medium apples, peeled, halved, cored, and cut into 1/2-inch wedges
- 1/4 cup packed Splenda Brown Sugar Blend
- 1/4 cup water
- 1 tablespoon lemon juice
- 2 tablespoons gluten-free baking mix
- 1 teaspoon ground cinnamon
- 1/8 teaspoon ground nutmeg (optional)
- 1/8 teaspoon salt

Topping
- 3/4 cup gluten-free baking mix, such as Bob's Red Mill
- 3 tablespoons canola oil
- 3 tablespoons water
- 2 teaspoons sugar
- 1/4 teaspoon ground cinnamon

1. Preheat the oven to 425°F.
2. Combine the filling ingredients in a medium bowl and toss until well coated. Place in 9-inch deep-dish pie pan.
3. In the same medium bowl, combine the 3/4 cup baking mix, oil, and water. Stir until well blended and sprinkle evenly over the apples by crumbling between your fingers. Bake 40–45 minutes or until crust is lightly browned.
4. In a small bowl, combine the 2 teaspoons sugar and 1/4 teaspoon cinnamon. Sprinkle evenly over the crust.

EXCHANGES/FOOD CHOICES		
2 Carbohydrate, 1 Fat	Cholesterol	0 mg
	Sodium	225 mg
	Potassium	180 mg
BASIC NUTRITIONAL VALUES:	Total Carbohydrate	27 g
Calories 165	Dietary Fiber	3 g
Calories from Fat 55	Sugars	11 g
Total Fat 6.0 g	Protein	2 g
Saturated Fat 0.4 g	Phosphorus	45 mg
Trans Fat 0.0 g		

PINEAPPLE PEACH OAT CRUMBLE

Serves 8 • Serving Size: 1/2 cup filling and about 2 tablespoons
topping • Makes about 4 cups fruit filling and about 1 cup crumble topping

---

Crumble

> 2 ounces chopped pecan pieces
> 1/2 cup gluten-free rolled oats
> 1/2 cup gluten-free corn or gluten-free Rice Chex-style cereal, crumbled
> 1/2 teaspoon ground cinnamon
> 1/4 teaspoon ground nutmeg
> 1/8 teaspoon salt
> 1 tablespoon canola oil
> 2 tablespoons packed Splenda Brown Sugar Blend

Base

> 2 8-ounce cans pineapple tidbits in own juice, undrained
> 1 pound frozen unsweetened peach slices, thawed and chopped
> 1 tablespoon cornstarch
> 2 tablespoons packed Splenda Brown Sugar Blend
> 1 1/2 tablespoons trans-fat-free margarine
> 1 teaspoon vanilla extract

---

1. In a medium mixing bowl, combine all crumble ingredients, except the oil and Splenda Brown Sugar Blend. Stir to blend thoroughly. Heat oil in a medium nonstick skillet over medium heat until hot. Tilt skillet to coat bottom evenly. Sprinkle oat mixture evenly over bottom of skillet, stir to blend, cook 2 minutes, stirring occasionally. Add the Splenda Brown Sugar Blend, and cook 1 minute or until slightly fragrant, but no longer than 1 minute, stirring constantly. Remove skillet from heat and place mixture on a separate plate.

2. To skillet, add the pineapple and its juice, peaches, and cornstarch. Stir until cornstarch is completely dissolved. Place over medium-high heat, bring to a boil, and continue to boil 2 minutes or until slightly thickened. Remove from heat, stir in Splenda Brown Sugar Blend, margarine, and vanilla, and top with crumble.

3. For peak flavors, let stand at least 2 hours to absorb flavors and blend. You can store this in the refrigerator for up to 3 days.

COOK'S TIP
Do not cook the topping any longer than recommended in directions, or else the topping will become very crunchy while it is cooling.

EXCHANGES/FOOD CHOICES
2 Carbohydrate, 1 1/2 Fat

BASIC NUTRITIONAL VALUES:

Calories	190
Calories from Fat	80
Total Fat	9.0 g
Saturated Fat	1.0 g
Trans Fat	0.0 g
Cholesterol	0 mg
Sodium	70 mg
Potassium	235 mg
Total Carbohydrate	28 g
Dietary Fiber	3 g
Sugars	16 g
Protein	2 g
Phosphorus	60 mg

SNEAKY Z BROWNIES

Serves 12 • Serving Size: 1 brownie and about 2 tablespoons whipped topping mixture • Makes 12 brownies and about 1 1/2 cups topping

Brownies
      Cooking spray
   1 16-ounce package gluten-free brownie mix
   1 medium zucchini, shredded
   2 tablespoons canola oil
   4 egg whites

Topping
   3 tablespoons gluten-free, lower sodium, 33%-less-sugar peanut butter, such as Jif
1 1/2 cups frozen sugar-free whipped topping, thawed

1. Preheat the oven to 325°F.
2. Lightly coat an 11-inch by 7-inch glass baking pan with cooking spray.
3. Combine the brownie mix, zucchini, oil, and egg whites in a medium bowl. Pour the batter into the baking pan and bake 30–35 minutes or until a wooden pick inserted 2 inches from edge comes out clean. Place pan on cooling rack to cool completely.
4. Place the peanut butter in a medium microwave-safe bowl and microwave on high for 30 seconds or until slightly melted. Fold in the whipped topping.
5. To serve, cut the brownies into 12 pieces and top each with equal amounts of the whipped topping mixture.

| COOK'S TIP | Refrigerate leftover brownies and the whipped topping mixture separately in airtight containers for up to 1 week. |

EXCHANGES/FOOD CHOICES
2 Carbohydrate, 1 Fat

BASIC NUTRITIONAL VALUES:

Calories	215
Calories from Fat	55
Total Fat	6.0 g
Saturated Fat	1.4 g
Trans Fat	0.0 g
Cholesterol	0 mg
Sodium	220 mg
Potassium	270 mg
Total Carbohydrate	32 g
Dietary Fiber	2 g
Sugars	18 g
Protein	4 g
Phosphorus	110 mg

OLD-TIME OATMEAL-RAISIN COOKIES

Serves 27 • Serving Size: 2 cookies • Makes 54 cookies

3/4	cup granulated sugar
1/4	cup packed Splenda Brown Sugar Blend
3/4	cup canola oil
2	large eggs
1 1/2	teaspoons vanilla, butter, and nut flavoring OR 2 teaspoons vanilla extract
1 1/2	cups gluten-free, all-purpose baking flour, such as Bob's Red Mill
1	tablespoon ground cinnamon
1/2	teaspoon ground nutmeg
3/4	teaspoon salt
1/2	teaspoon baking soda
3	cups gluten-free rolled oats
1 1/4	cups raisins
	Cooking spray

1. Preheat oven to 350°F.
2. In a medium bowl, combine the sugar, Splenda Brown Sugar Blend, and oil. Using an electric mixer, beat on medium-high speed 1 minute. Add the eggs and vanilla. Beat until well blended.
3. In another medium bowl, stir together the flour, cinnamon, nutmeg, salt, and baking soda. Add the flour mixture to the wet ingredients and beat on medium speed until well blended. Add oats and beat until well blended. Stir in the raisins.
4. Drop slightly rounded tablespoons of cookie dough onto a nonstick cookie sheet lightly coated with cooking spray. Bake for 8 minutes, or until puffed and lightly brown on bottom. (They may not appear to be done at this point but will continue to cook while cooling. Do not cook until the edges are brown because it will be too dry.) Cool 1 minute on baking sheet and then transfer to wire rack. Continue with remaining cookie dough.

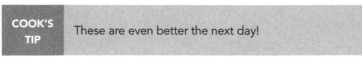

COOK'S TIP	These are even better the next day!

EXCHANGES/FOOD CHOICES
1 1/2 Carbohydrate, 1 1/2 Fat

BASIC NUTRITIONAL VALUES:

Calories	175
Calories from Fat	65
Total Fat	7.0 g
Saturated Fat	0.7 g
Trans Fat	0.0 g
Cholesterol	15 mg
Sodium	95 mg
Potassium	125 mg
Total Carbohydrate	25 g
Dietary Fiber	2 g
Sugars	11 g
Protein	3 g
Phosphorus	80 mg

QUINOA COOKIE BALLS

Serves 25 • Serving Size: 2 balls • Makes about 50 balls

KID FRIENDLY

1/2	cup dry quinoa
1 1/4	cups water
1/2	cup low-sodium, 33%-less-sugar peanut butter
1/4	cup honey
1	ripe medium banana, mashed
1/2	cup flaked sweetened coconut
1 1/2	cups quick-cooking oats
1/4	cup ground flax meal
1	teaspoon ground cinnamon
1/2	teaspoon salt
1/3	cup mini chocolate chips

1. Preheat oven to 350°F.

2. In a small saucepan, bring the water to a boil over high heat. Stir in quinoa, reduce heat, cover, and simmer 12 minutes. Drain in a fine-mesh sieve and run under cold water to cool completely. Shake off excess liquid.

3. In a medium bowl, stir together the quinoa, peanut butter, honey, banana, and coconut until well blended. In another medium bowl, combine the oats, flax, cinnamon, and salt. Add the quinoa mixture and chocolate chips. Stir until well blended.

4. Using a tablespoon, roll into 1-inch balls and place on a greased cookie sheet. Bake for 10 minutes, until cookies are browned on the bottom. Remove from the oven. Cool completely on cookie sheet. Refrigerate leftovers in an airtight container for up to 1 week.

EXCHANGES/FOOD CHOICES		Cholesterol	0 mg
1 Carbohydrate, 1 Fat		Sodium	65 mg
		Potassium	120 mg
BASIC NUTRITIONAL VALUES:		Total Carbohydrate	14 g
Calories	110	Dietary Fiber	2 g
Calories from Fat	45	Sugars	6 g
Total Fat	5.0 g	Protein	3 g
Saturated Fat	1.5 g	Phosphorus	75 mg
Trans Fat	0.0 g		

BERRY CUSTARD CUPS

Serves 6 • Serving Size: 1/2 cup custard and 1/3 cup berries •
Makes 3 cups custard and 2 cups berries

---

    3 cups fat-free evaporated milk
  1/2 cup egg substitute
  1/4 cup cornstarch
  1/4 teaspoon salt
  1/3 cup packed Splenda Brown Sugar Blend
    1 teaspoon vanilla, butter, and nut flavoring OR 1 1/2 teaspoons vanilla
       extract
    2 cups quartered strawberries or blueberries

---

1. In a medium saucepan, whisk together the milk, egg substitute, cornstarch, and salt until cornstarch is dissolved. Cook over medium heat until thickened, stirring frequently. Bring to a boil, boil 1 minute, stirring constantly with a whisk. Remove from heat.

2. Stir in the sugar and vanilla, butter, and nut flavoring. Pour into 6 ramekins and refrigerate until set. Serve topped with berries.

EXCHANGES/FOOD CHOICES		
1 Fat-Free Milk, 1 1/2 Carbohydrate	Cholesterol	5 mg
	Sodium	285 mg
	Potassium	545 mg
BASIC NUTRITIONAL VALUES:	Total Carbohydrate	34 g
Calories	190	Dietary Fiber	1 g
Calories from Fat	0	Sugars	22 g
Total Fat	0.0 g	Protein	12 g
Saturated Fat	0.2 g	Phosphorus	265 mg
Trans Fat	0.0 g		

PB BANANA STUFFED COOKIES

Serves 4 • Serving Size: 2 cookies • Makes 8 stuffed cookies

2	tablespoons low-sodium, 33%-less-sugar peanut butter
2	tablespoons nonfat plain Greek yogurt
1	small banana, cut in 24 slices total
16	gluten-free gingersnap cookies (3 1/3 ounces total; 6 grams each)

1. In a small bowl, stir together the peanut butter and yogurt. Spoon equal amounts on the flat side of each cookie. Place 3 banana slices on top of 8 cookies, top with the remaining 8 cookies, and press down gently to adhere. Serve immediately or wrap in foil and freeze until needed.

EXCHANGES/FOOD CHOICES
1 1/2 Carbohydrate, 1 1/2 Fat

BASIC NUTRITIONAL VALUES:

Calories	185
Calories from Fat	80
Total Fat	9.0 g
Saturated Fat	0.9 g
Trans Fat	0.0 g
Cholesterol	0 mg
Sodium	85 mg
Potassium	310 mg
Total Carbohydrate	24 g
Dietary Fiber	2 g
Sugars	13 g
Protein	4 g
Phosphorus	90 mg

COFFEEHOUSE CHOCOLATE-CHERRY FREEZE

Serves 8 • Serving Size: 1 slice • Makes one 8-inch pie

- 4 cups gluten-free, fat-free, sugar-free vanilla or chocolate ice cream, such as Blue Bunny
- 2 teaspoons instant coffee granules
- 8 ounces frozen unsweetened dark sweet cherries, partially thawed, and halved
- 2 ounces gluten-free whipped topping, such as Reddi-wip
- 1 1/2 ounces slivered almonds, toasted

---

1. Spoon the ice cream into 8-inch round cake or pie pan. Sprinkle evenly with the coffee granules, arrange the cherries on top. Spoon the whipped topping evenly over all and sprinkle with the almonds. Cover and freeze until firm.

EXCHANGES/FOOD CHOICES		Cholesterol	10 mg
2 Carbohydrate, 1/2 Fat		Sodium	70 mg
		Potassium	280 mg
BASIC NUTRITIONAL VALUES:		Total Carbohydrate	28 g
Calories	155	Dietary Fiber	6 g
Calories from Fat	35	Sugars	10 g
Total Fat	4.0 g	Protein	6 g
Saturated Fat	0.9 g	Phosphorus	90 mg
Trans Fat	0.0 g		

COOKIE-CRUMBLE ICE CREAM CUPS

Serves 4 • Serving Size: 1/2 cup • Makes 2 cups

KID FRIENDLY

2 cups gluten-free, fat-free, sugar-free vanilla or chocolate
   ice cream, such as Blue Bunny
4 gluten-free chocolate sandwich cookies (1 3/4 ounces total;
   12 grams each), coarsely crumbled
4 teaspoons sugar-free caramel ice cream topping
1 ounce slivered almonds, toasted and coarsely chopped

1. Place the ice cream in a medium bowl. Add the cookie crumbs and gently
   stir together until just blended. Spoon into four 6-ounce ramekins. Spoon
   equal amounts of the ice cream topping on each and sprinkle evenly with
   the nuts.
2. Cover with foil and freeze until firm, about 4 hours.

COOK'S TIP	A variation: Stir all of the ingredients together until just blended and freeze in frozen-pop molds for a fun treat!

EXCHANGES/FOOD CHOICES
2 Carbohydrate, 1 Fat

BASIC NUTRITIONAL VALUES:

Calories	190
Calories from Fat	55
Total Fat	6.0 g
Saturated Fat	0.4 g
Trans Fat	0.0 g
Cholesterol	5 mg
Sodium	110 mg
Potassium	295 mg
Total Carbohydrate	34 g
Dietary Fiber	6 g
Sugars	11 g
Protein	6 g
Phosphorus	115 mg

Appendix
Celiac Disease Resources

ORGANIZATIONS

American Celiac Disease Alliance
www.americanceliac.org

Celiac Disease Foundation
www.celiac.org

Celiac Sprue Association
www.csaceliacs.org

Gluten Intolerance Group
www.gluten.net

National Foundation for Celiac Awareness
www.celiaccentral.org

CELIAC EDUCATION AND RESEARCH CENTERS

University of Chicago Celiac Disease Program
www.cureceliacdisease.org

Celiac Disease Center at Columbia University Medical Center
www.celiacdiseasecenter.columbia.edu

Celiac Center Beth Israel Deaconess Medical Center
www.celiacnow.org

BOOKS

Case S: *Gluten-Free Diet: A Comprehensive Resource Guide.*
Regina, Saskatchewan, Canada, Case Nutrition Consulting, Inc., 2010

Green PHR, Jones R: *Celiac Disease: A Hidden Epidemic.* New York,
William Morrow, 2010

Koeller K, La France R: *Let's Eat Out with Celiac/Coeliac and Food Allergies!
Reference for Gluten and Allergy Free Diets.* Chicago, IL, Gluten Free Passport,
2011

Korn D: *Kids with Celiac Disease: A Family Guide to Raising Happy, Healthy,
Gluten-Free Children.* Bethesda, MD, Woodbine House, 2001

Thompson T: *American Dietetic Association Easy Gluten-Free: Expert Nutrition
Advice with More than 100 Recipes.* Hoboken, NJ, Wiley, 2010

Thompson T: *The Gluten-Free Nutrition Guide.* New York, McGraw-Hill, 2008

EATING OUT RESOURCES

Websites and Phone Apps

Allergy Eats!
www.allergyeats.com

Find Me Gluten Free
www.findmeglutenfree.com

The Celiac Scene
www.theceliacscene.com

Gluten-Free Allergy Free Passport
www.glutenfreepassport.com

Triumph Dining
www.triumphdining.com

Gluten-Free Restaurant Awareness Program
www.glutenfreerestaurants.org

WEBSITES AND MAGAZINES

www.glutenfreeliving.com
Magazine and website that provide practical, reliable information about the gluten-free diet.

www.livebetteramerica.com/health/gluten-free
Live Better America is a community and e-commerce site developed and owned by General Mills, Inc.

www.livingwithout.com
Magazine and website for people living with food allergies and sensitivities.

REFERENCES

Academy of Nutrition and Dietetics Evidence Analysis Library: Evidence-based nutrition practice guideline on diabetes 1 and 2, 2008. Available at www.adaevidencelibrary.com. Accessed 1 October 2012

American Diabetes Association: Standards of medical care in diabetes—2013. *Diabetes Care* 36 (Suppl. 1):S11–S66, 2013

American Diabetes Association: Standards of medical care in diabetes—2012. *Diabetes Care* 35 (Suppl. 1):S11–S49, 2012

American Dietetic Association Evidence Analysis Library: Evidence-based nutrition practice guideline on celiac disease, 2009. Available at www.adaevidencelibrary.com. Accessed 1 October 2012

Case S: *Gluten-Free Diet: A Comprehensive Resource Guide.* Regina, Saskatchewan, Canada, Case Nutrition Consulting, Inc., 2010

Glycemic Index website. Available at www.glycemicindex.com. Accessed 1 October 2012

Green P, Jones R: *Celiac Disease: A Hidden Epidemic.* New York, Harper Collins, 2010

Kupper C, Higgins L: Combining diabetes and gluten-free management guidelines. *Pract Gastroenterol* XXXI:68–83, March 2007

Marchese A, Lovati E, Biagi F, Corazza GR: Celiac disease and type 1 diabetes: epidemiological, clinical implications, and effects of gluten-free diet. *Endocrine* 43:1–2, 2013

Rondinelli L: *The How and Why of Celiac Disease and Diabetes.* Available at www.dlife.com/diabetes/associated_conditions/celiac_disease/lara_rondinelli/celiac-disease-test. Accessed 1 October 2012

Rubio-Tapia A, Ludvigsson JF, Brantner TL, Murray JA, Everhart JE: The prevalence of celiac disease in the United States. *Am J Gastroenterol* 107:1538–1544, 2012

Schuppan D, Hahn E: Celiac disease and its link to type 1 diabetes mellitus. *J Pediatr Endocrinol Metab* 14 (Suppl. 1):597–605, 2001

Schwarzenberg J, Brunzell C: Type 1 diabetes and celiac disease: overview and medical nutrition therapy. *Diabetes Spectrum* 15:197–201, 2001

Thompson T, Simpson S: *Counting Gluten-Free Carbohydrates: A dietitian resource for counseling individuals with diabetes and celiac disease.* Available at www.csaceliacs.info/files.jsp?file_id=11. Accessed 1 October 2012

University of Chicago Celiac Disease Center website. Available at www.cureceliacdisease.org. Accessed 1 October 2012

University of Chicago Celiac Disease Center. *Jump Start Your Gluten-Free Diet.* Chicago, IL, R & R Publishing, 2013

Whole Grains Council website. Available at www.wholegrainscouncil.org. Accessed 1 October 2012

Index